Awaken Holistic Medicine Knowledge for Beginners: Secrets to Naturally Heal and Balance Your Body With Herbal Remedies

Imagine Having Secret Herbs in the Palm of Your Hand: Look Inside

Arden Dagon

advice. The content within this book has been derived from various sources. Please consult a licensed professional before attempting any techniques outlined in this book.

By reading this document, the reader agrees that under no circumstances is the author responsible for any losses, direct or indirect, that are incurred as a result of the use of the information contained within this document, including, but not limited to, errors, omissions, or inaccuracies.

Table of Contents

Introduction

The fact that you are reading this book confirms one thing: that you are beginning to wake up to the illusion of modern healthcare. We, as a species, have transitioned from rich cultural traditions, natural medicine, and a connection with nature to a mass-produced, commercialized society. A society that is not built for you to thrive. Commerce and profit are placed on a higher pedestal than your health. The world where we currently reside makes it *so* difficult to maintain good health, with processed and toxin-laced foods lining the shelves in every store. The need for convenience and low prices has facilitated a transition from food to "food-like" products. These genetically modified foods masquerade as the real deal, but lurking behind the first bite lies an unsavory truth. Dietary factors are now the cause of 22% of all adult deaths. It's certainly terrifying to think that food, something that's meant to keep us alive, could actually be killing us.

Whatever your reason is for reading this book, whether you are trying to heal a particular disease, reduce stress, or just improve your general health, you have made an excellent first step. As modern medicine routinely fails, society has begun to seek out traditional ailments from years gone by as a solution to all kinds of illnesses.

Long before the scientific revolution provided us with the medicine and pills that we use to treat illness today, humans looked to natural sources to fight sickness and disease. Herbal and holistic medicine has been used in every culture throughout history. Holistic medicine sees a melting pot of ancient wisdom, potent herbs, and energetics all come together to heal the body naturally. Who would have thought that vibrant, colorful spices, earthy funghi, and fragrant herbs could be the key to optimal health? Traditional medicine not only encourages the use of these natural wonders, but also places them as the foundation of achieving true holistic health. The biomolecular effects of herbs have been shown to protect against oxidative stress, inflammation, disease, and even aging.

As you combine secret herbal combinations with the ancient knowledge, you will learn in this book to embrace a new reality. A reality where you are no longer a slave to chemicals. Where you eat food that heals you, instead of poisoning you. Where instead of inevitably facing mental and physical disease and discomfort, you thrive with a sense of energetic passion.

How am I so confident about this? I am living proof. I have achieved optimal health, avoiding any food and environmental allergies in my body for over 25 years. My journey started at a young age when I discovered alternative health. I was completely spellbound by all of the amazing information that exists. From ancient Indian Ayurveda to traditional Chinese medicine. It's amazing to me that these wonderful insights have been almost completely discarded, in place of laboratory-created chemicals and 'fake' foods. Over the 25 years that I studied alternative health, I collated life-changing information on how to create the ultimate healthy, energetic version of myself, living with almost zero toxins. In addition to looking younger, revitalized, and more vibrant, I feel incredible.

The key to transforming your health begins with awareness. Once you master awareness of your current situation, you can then begin to change your habits. By changing your habits, you will change your reality and your health. It's never too late to start. All you need is a strong determination and the powerful knowledge that is packed into this book.

Throughout this book, we will explore the ancient traditional medicine that outdates the contemporary medicine used worldwide today. Learning about the roots of holistic medicine will allow you to see how this form of treatment originated and became as popular as it was today. Holistic medicine dates back over 5,000 years, with a rich history across many cultures. Before we had surgeries and pills, society looked to natural causes for healing. Many of these treatments were so successful that they are still used to this day and age across the world. You will learn the powerful effect that these treatments can have on your health. Whether you want to heal a condition, or just experience better overall well-being, understanding the history of holistic medicine will provide some much needed context for you.

Although it is often overlooked, the air that we breathe is a huge contributing factor to our overall health. With pollution rife in our society, it's crucial that you understand the main risks to your respiratory system.

You'll be educated on the top pollutants and the effects that each of them will have on your body. Knowledge is power, understanding the risks will help you to avoid them.

One of the main pillars of holistic health is what you eat. The food system that we're given access to is rigged against us, knowing this will open your mind to an incredible alternative–organic, whole foods. You will discover what food you need to avoid, and what food you should start to eat in abundance. I have also included major red flags in food, such as food groups that you should never consume, and what foods are the most genetically modified.

Beyond your body, your mindset plays a huge role in your overall health. Unlike contemporary medicine, holistic healing takes into account your mental and emotional health, too. Mastering these will have instant positive effects on your physical health. You will uncover all of the areas of your life that you'll need to work on to create true emotional well-being. You'll be so surprised at how quickly your physical health could improve by just working on your mindset.

A huge part of holistic healing is herbal medicine. This can be something that is so overwhelming to a beginner. With so much conflicting information, and many internet sources existing simply to deter you from trying it, it can be hard to find reliable information. I have provided a full guide to getting started with holistic and herbal medicine. In an attempt to be as unbiased as possible, you will also find the advantages and disadvantages of herbal medicine, so that you can make an informed decision as to whether you would like to try it. As finding reliable sources is difficult, I'll also let you in on the best ways to identify trustworthy sources of information so that you can continue your own research.

From there, you'll learn all of the different methods to consume herbal medicine. You might want to experiment with all of them to find out what one is best for you. I've listed the most popular methods, including instructions on how you can make them yourself at home. Although you can embark on the majority of your holistic healing journey independently, it's great to rope in the authority of a licensed holistic doctor. You'll find a chapter on how to identify and assess holistic doctors, including all the questions that you need to ask them. The knowledge in this book, teamed with a professional, will provide you with the ultimate armor against ill health.

This book has four sections to help you to navigate it in a simple and efficient way. Each section has a description of what you can expect to learn in the subsequent chapters. Simply navigate to each section to discover what you will learn in the chapters for that particular section.

I believe in you, all you need to succeed on your journey to optimum health now is the determination and perseverance not to fail. Remain open minded, positive, and ready, and you will step into the healthiest version of yourself.

Section 1:

The Beginning Is the Ending

In this section, you will begin your voyage into what holistic health is and all that it has to offer. Your current view of your health and the modern medical system will be shaken, with shocking truths revealed to you with hard-hitting evidence. With an introduction to what holistic health is and the history and origins of its influential philosophies, you will become an expert in all things holistic.

Chapter 1:

The History of Holistic Medicine

To truly understand how you can use holistic medicine to transform your life, it's helpful to explore its history and define exactly what it is. Holistic medicine can be traced back thousands of years, with roots that span many different cultures. The term 'holism' itself was coined by Smuts in 1926, aiming to conceptualize humans as greater than the sum of their parts. This holistic approach is vastly different from the modern doctor's office visit. In today's society, when you visit a doctor, they are primarily concerned with treating symptoms as opposed to uncovering the reason for the illness. With the "in and out" attitude of many of today's modern practitioners, it's no wonder the doctors aren't considering your overall health. To better understand how you can get started with holistic healing, you're probably curious as to where it originated in the first place. Holistic healing predates any of the medicine that's stocked on conventional pharmacist's shelves and the cures peddled in modern science books. This wonderful, age-old wisdom is accessible to you immediately, all you have to do is open your mind to learning about it. To begin, let's explore the definition and meaning of exactly what holistic medicine is.

Defining Holistic Medicine

The American Holistic Health Association (AHHA) describes holistic health as an approach that considers the whole person and how that person interacts with their environment. It looks beyond the identification of symptoms and recognizes the connection of mind, body, and spirit in achieving optimum well-being. True well-being comes from everything functioning at its best simultaneously. The ultimate goal according to holistic philosophy is optimum health through proper balance in life.

In terms of holistic medicine, practitioners see the body as being made up of several interdependent parts, much like a machine. If one of these parts does not work properly, it, in turn, affects all of the other parts. Using this logic, you can see how when we have an imbalance in our physical, mental, or spiritual self, it negatively impacts all other areas. This in turn wreaks havoc on your overall health.

In stark contrast to mainstream healthcare, holistic medicine steers away from the use of drugs and surgery as the first defensive structures. Instead, holistic medicine favors treatments such as:

- Modifications to your diet
- Incorporating exercise into your daily routine

- Improving your environment
- Making modifications to your behaviors and attitudes
- Counseling or coaching in areas such as relationships and spirituality
- Bioenergy enhancements

These treatments are not only non-invasive and arguably safer than medicine and surgery, but they also address the root problem. Rather than dismissing an illness as simply the presentation of symptoms, holistic medicine dives deep into where the illness itself originated. Our bodies are powerful mechanisms that have the incredible ability to heal themselves. The aim of working with these holistic treatments is to harness this power, improving the flow of life-force energy or *prana* in your body.

One interesting aspect of holistic philosophy and holistic medicine is that it hands the responsibility over to the patient. In mainstream medicine, a patient will consult a doctor, desperately seeking answers to their health woes. The responsibility is almost entirely placed on the doctor, with the expectation that they know to solve the patient's problems. This one-way form of treatment sees the patient relying solely on the advice and medicine provided by the doctor. Holistic medicine takes an entirely different approach. According to the AHHA, holistic medicine teaches patients to become responsible for their health. The benefits of doing so include receiving therapeutic benefits in a cost-effective way, better treatment of chronic disease, and the creation of optimum health.

With holistic medicine, there is no longer the need to adhere to long surgery waiting times or to painstakingly take medicine in the hope that it might just work. Holistic medicine allows you to feel empowered and take back control, optimizing your health on your terms.

The History of Holistic Medicine

It's crucial to learn about the history of holistic medicine and understand a little more about where it came from. This incredible school of thought dates back over 5000 years, far before the emergence of Western (allopathic) medicine. Holistic healing itself can be traced back to some of history's earliest civilizations. Dating back to prehistoric times, when plants and herbs were used to heal wounds, holistic healing spans millennia.

Greece 400 BC

A notable era for holistic medicine is 400 BC when Hippocrates identified a revolutionary schema where natural (as opposed to supernatural) explanations were provided for illness and disease. Before this, illness was almost always associated with spiritual causes. Demons and deities were thought of as the culprit for seizures, which supposedly occurred due to the gods being angered. Hippocrates theorized that illnesses resulted in imbalances in the body's 'humor.' These were blood, black bile, yellow bile, and phlegm or mucus. Practitioners were encouraged to advise patients on how to restore humoral balance, bringing them back to health. This theory of balancing the different parts of the body became the basis for holistic health philosophy.

Following Hippocrates, Galen, a Roman anatomist discovered a link between our emotions and illness. He proposed a direct relationship between a patient's body and mind, noticing illness occurring after an emotional shock. This built upon the idea of balancing the body, extending the concept to the mental and spiritual self too.

China 1600 BC

Traditional Chinese medicine (TCM) was created almost 5000 years ago, making it one of the oldest forms of holistic medicine that there is. It was weaved into Confucius' philosophies and some of the oldest Chinese texts that there are. TCM identified the interconnectivity of the body, viewing it as a small universe of connected systems. It also noted life force energy or *qi* and how it plays a role in overall health.

As opposed to the unified nation that it is today, China was historically composed of several different dynasties. Each had its ruler and as a result, had access to different teachers and views. This led to somewhat of a conflict amongst theories, as knowledge was based on contributions from each particular dynasty alone. Therefore, practitioners from alternate dynasties may have prescribed a patient a different remedy for the same ailment.

TCM conceptualized the human body with reference to the universe. They likened the skin of the human body to the texture of the earth's ground, and our internal organs to wood, fire, water, earth, and metal. The idea was that no being could exist without a connection to its environment. These concepts formed the basis of Taoism, which helped to shape TCM based on the belief that everything in the universe is interdependent. TCM highlighted the fact that the body is an organic whole, as opposed to lots of separate parts. All of the body's individual parts are reliant on each other, with each part of the body somehow relating to our organs.

TCM spread to Western countries from the sixteenth century; however, only a handful of the practices remain relevant in Western society. The range of disciplines under the TCM umbrella includes acupuncture, cupping, herbs, meditation, and *tai chi*. The aim of these treatments is often to encourage and maintain the flow of *qi* in the body. Rather than taking a targeted approach to pinpoint and treat specific symptoms, the idea behind TCM treatments is that they are designed to restore the balance of the whole body.

India 2500 BC

Another ancient source of wisdom can be traced back to India. In the *Vedas,* which are sacred Indian books, writing can be found on holistic medicine. The most relevant of these, the *Atharvaveda* contains the origins of

Ayurveda. This traditional Indian medicine system is based on balance and moderation. As one of the oldest care systems, there is, Ayurveda seeks to synthesize mind, body, and spirit. As opposed to using medicine, it seeks to restore body balance through eating well, breathwork, sleeping well, and creating a relaxing environment. In Ayurvedic practice, good food is seen as medicine and the path to enhanced health, as well as strengthening the connection between mind and body. This healing method focuses on seven constituent body elements and three biological energies called *doshas*.

Everyone has their own personal mind and body composition or *dosha*. Doshas encompass the five elements and depend on other factors such as the planetary alignment and the food that your parents ate before you were conceived. Each one of us has a mix of all three doshas which are *Vata, Pitta,* and *Kapha*. However, we tend to have one primary dosha that is predominant and known as *prakruti*. You may have a mix of two dominant doshas, or rarely, a balanced mix of all three.

Due to external factors such as your emotional stability, the food that you eat, and your sleep habits, imbalance or *vikruti* can form in the body. The idea is that through Ayurvedic practice, you restore your balance and move back to a natural way of life. In terms of the functions of each of the doshas, *Vata* is responsible for catabolism, *Pitta* governs metabolism, and *Kapha* manages anabolism. Any form of imbalance between them is thought to be the cause of illness, sickness, and disease. To balance and rejuvenate the body, Ayurveda utilizes the *pancha karma* approach. This uses five actions to remove toxins from the body. A build-up of toxins prevents life force energy from being able to flow correctly, which also leads to illness. By cleansing the mind and body of these clogging toxins, life force energy is freed, flowing throughout the body to create wellbeing and vitality. This highlights the ancient Indian's view that whole-body harmony is needed to be truly healthy.

Seeing the body as a whole is the crucial theory that underpins all holistic health philosophies. As you can see, throughout history this is the commonality that has transcended cultures. Knowing a little more about the background history of holistic health will arm you with the information needed when you're conducting your research on herbal medicine. Now that you're confident on exactly what holistic medicine entails, you can begin to peel back the layers of all of the components that make up true holistic healthy living.

Section 2:

The Basics of Why People Get Sick

In this section, you'll uncover why people get sick in the first place. There are countless ways in which you can develop a sickness or disease. In contrast to what the media will have you believe, disease is not just due to hereditary conditions or bad luck. Your environment, the air that you breathe, the food that you eat, and even the thoughts that you think all have the potential to make you sick. The first step in protecting yourself is to understand all the different ways in which you can become ill. The chapters in this section will provide you with a rich education on all of the ways that you can get sick so that you can build your defenses against them.

Chapter 2:

The First Imbalance Is

People's Physical Body

If the literature surrounding holistic health and why you get sick all points to imbalance, you may be wondering where exactly this begins. The first imbalance is in your physical body. These imbalances can either be internal or external. One of the most common external factors for illness in holistic health philosophy is the interaction of your body with the environment. As we move away from picturesque societies featuring roads littered with green trees and natural foliage, instead sky-high buildings, man-made chemicals, and pollutants replace the oxygen-rich air we once used to breathe. This new environment that we have created poses vast risks to our physical bodies. The simple act of stepping out of your front door confronts you with an attack of harmful chemicals. Throughout this chapter, you will identify some of the most common pollutants so that you can recognize and protect yourself against them.

Air pollutants are the silent, yet deadly killers that you may not have ever even considered. The toxins in air pollution can slowly poison, or in some rare cases, instantly kill you. Our respiratory system is constantly under attack daily. As much as we would all love to believe that oxygen is the only gas we breathe, the truth is far from this. The mix of multiple gasses that now exists in our air affects everything from our blood, respiratory and cardiovascular systems. These covert killers lurk in the air and wreak havoc on your health. They are also associated with oxidative stress and inflammation in human cells. It doesn't require a degree in science to recognize that pollutants are something that you should make yourself aware of. The following pollutants are the most well-known and dangerous.

Air Pollution

As we explored previously, air pollution is a deadly and unavoidable phenomenon. The most common form of air pollution, traffic-related air pollution (TRAP), is a form of pollution that results from motor vehicle emissions. The fossil fuel combustion in the engines of these vehicles has been linked to cardiovascular disease and impaired child development. In urban cities, this type of pollution is at its worst, becoming almost unavoidable. One frightening factor regarding this toxin is that it causes complications in more than 10% of pregnancies worldwide and is one of the leading causes of fetal deaths.

Ozone

Another dangerous gas creating issues in your body is ozone (O3). This is an extremely reactive gas comprised of three oxygen atoms that occurs in the Earth's atmosphere. This gas occurs both naturally, and as a result of man-made creation. When inhaled, it creates a chemical reaction in the respiratory tract which creates several serious issues for your health.

Noxious Gasses

We can categorize gasses that are harmful to humans as noxious gasses, these gasses can be extremely dangerous not only to humans but to all living things. Often, these gasses build up in workspaces that are not properly ventilated. Noxious gasses such as hydrogen sulfide, which causes loss of smell, carbon monoxide, which can slowly kill, and solvents, which can cause the nervous system to shut down, are highly toxic.

Particulate Matter

Any solid or liquid particles that are found in the air are known as particle matter. These particles are typically invisible, however, some are visible to the naked eye, such as dirt, dust, and soot. Several of these particles are formed as the result of chemical reactions between noxious gasses. Other instances see particle matter emitted from construction, fires, or natural disasters. When the particle matter is inhaled, it causes chaos in our system. Particles that are less than 2.5 micrometers are regarded as the worst for your health, with the ability to get deep into your lungs and even your bloodstream.

Volatile Organic Compounds

Don't let the term 'organic' in the name fool you, volatile organic compounds or "VOC" are extremely toxic. These gasses contain carbon and are often given off by strong materials such as glue, pesticide, cleaning products, and paint. Gasoline and petrol are also VOCs and can be highly dangerous when inhaled during combustion. These gasses turn to vapor on or around room temperature.

Carcinogens

Any substance that can cause cancer is known as a carcinogen. These can either be naturally occurring, such as the sun's UV rays, or viruses, or manmade, such as cigarettes or vehicle fumes. These substances sneak their way into your cell's DNA and produce mutations, which in turn cause cancer. It's hugely important to identify carcinogens so that you can limit your exposure to them. In recent years, scientists have discovered that everything from asbestos, to processed meat, are carcinogens. It is important to note, however, that not everyone who has exposure to a carcinogen will get cancer. However, limiting your exposure to them will in turn reduce your risk of cancer.

The Respiratory System

Your respiratory system is working every day to keep you alive. This intricate network of tissue and organ helps you to breathe, absorbing oxygen and dispelling carbon dioxide and other waste gasses from your system. Several different internal parts make up the respiratory system, including the mouth and nose, lungs, throat, sinuses, trachea, and bronchial tubes. The clever respiratory system is the reason that you're able to inhale and exhale, talk, smell, and deliver oxygen to your cells.

Breathing is more scientifically known as pulmonary ventilation. In pulmonary ventilation, the air is inhaled through the nose and mouth, moving through the larynx, and into the lungs. Following on from this, a phenomenon called external respiration then exchanges gasses between the lungs and blood. This is where the oxygen is swapped out for carbon dioxide waste gas. Finally, internal respiration occurs and gasses are exchanged between the tissues and bloodstream. Oxygen is transported into your cells, and waste carbon dioxide is promptly removed from them.

As this complex process occurs constantly, external threats to your respiratory system such as air pollutants are always ready to attack. Breathing in these pollutants can create severe problems for your health, such as heart attacks, cancer, and even premature death. The top cause of cancer is a result of respiratory pollutants. They should not be taken lightly when looking to defend yourself from disease.

The Cardiovascular System

Another important system to examine in terms of holistic health is your cardiovascular system. The cardiovascular system is responsible for transporting oxygen around the body and removing the waste, following on from the purpose of the respiratory system. For your body to receive all of the nutrients that it requires to run in tip-top condition, the cardiovascular system is essential.

The cardiovascular system itself is made up of your heart and a deep network of blood vessels that transport oxygen to your body. It also removes toxins and waste products from your body, disposing of anything that it doesn't need. No matter what time of the day, whether you're awake at your work desk, or fast asleep in bed, your incredible cardiovascular system will be working overtime to pump blood throughout your body. On average, your heart circulates 2,000 gallons of blood per day.

To circulate your blood, the cardiovascular system uses two circulation processes. The first is pulmonary circulation, this is where blood without oxygen floods into the right side of your heart. This blood is then directed to the lungs to fill itself up with oxygen and dispose of carbon dioxide. After it's been pumped up and oxidized, it comes back in through the left side of your heart. Ensuing this, systematic circulation occurs, where the blood that has received oxygen through the lungs then flows through the rest of the body. This provides oxygen to all of the cells in your body before the cycle starts again.

When it comes to pollutants, they directly affect the cardiovascular system, as they enter the bloodstream. Now that you know the delicate process that occurs and how the cardiovascular system cleans the blood of waste products, you can see how dangerous it is when toxic substances interfere. When we inhale toxic pollutants, they enter the blood and end up being transported through the bloodstream to all of our organs.

Cancer

Arguably the most devastating disease of all, cancer is a disease where cells grow uncontrollably and begin spreading to other parts of the body. Typically, our cells grow and multiply as a result of cell division, forming new cells as and when the body needs them. When normal cells are damaged or become old, they die and are replaced with new cells. Rarely, this seamless process encounters an error, and abnormal cells continue to expand and multiply when they aren't meant to. This causes tumors to form, which can either be benign, or cancerous.

Cancerous tumors can invade nearby tissue and create new tumors. These tumors create a path of destruction, stopping normal cells from growing when they encounter them. They also can tell blood vessels to grow towards them, supplying them with oxygen and removing waste in the same way that the circulatory system does. Cancer forms a genetic disease, with the changes in our genes altering the way that the cells function and grow. These genetic alterations often occur due to the DNA being damaged by external pollutants and carcinogens in the environment.

Every day, we inhale enough toxins and germs to cause a multitude of diseases. However, we don't contract every single disease that we are exposed to. Our bodies have excellent defense systems, and when properly trained and looked after, our bodies can strengthen themselves against the results of these toxic pollutants. Cancer develops throughout the body because when we inhale air pollutants, our respiratory and cardiovascular systems circulate the hazardous gasses around our bodies. When they are unable to filter out properly, they end up spreading to all of our organs and creating disease.

The key to defending yourself against these pollutants is to recognize the problem before you can solve it. These toxic pollutants can have either immediate or long-term detrimental effects on your health. Not only do they affect each system that they come into contact with, but they also affect the entire body, creating the need for holistic medicine and healing as it takes the whole body into account. Although you can't live in a bubble and avoid all of these issues, it's great to be able to identify them so that you can take small steps to protect yourself. Making small changes like ceasing use of air fresheners and other toxic pollutants is a great first step. I would recommend trying to expose yourself to fresh, clean air as often as possible. Whether it's taking a break from your work desk for a quick stroll outside, or a longer trip away to breathe fresh air from nature, your body will certainly thank you.

Chapter 3:

The Second Imbalance Is

People's Eating Habits

Toxic gas inhalation is not the sole culprit of society's health woes. Humans can enjoy an abundance of food and drink daily, however, food is not what it used to be. Food-like products line the shelves, laden with additives, colorings, and toxic chemicals that offer harm as opposed to health. Chain supermarkets are overfilled with processed, snack, and convenience food, but lacking in good-quality organic fruits and vegetables. The sad truth is that we have long forgotten the hunter-gatherer way of life that our ancestors pioneered. It's not all bad, however–organic natural food is making a comeback, with local stores offering an alternative to GMO grub.

When you're able to source organic produce from local shops, or even better–grow your own, you take back control of your health. As the masses awaken to the knowledge that healthy food is vital to a long life, consumer demand for organic goods has skyrocketed. Organic produce is now available in 3 out of 4 conventional grocery stores in the US. However, high premium prices currently remain despite the demand expansion. Don't let the high price point put you off, the money that you invest into buying good quality fruit and vegetables will save you thousands in medical bills down the line.

As we explored in the previous chapter, pesticides are one of the leading carcinogenic toxins found in modern society. As pesticides are used in traditional non-organic farming, you must seek out organic produce that does not use pesticides. You may also want to wash your produce in apple cider vinegar to ensure that any toxins that it has encountered on its journey into your home are removed.

Food and Drink Imbalances

As with all other areas of holistic health, ill-health all comes back to imbalance. An imbalance in the body can be created by eating certain types of food. Sugary, salty, sour, spicy, and bitter foods all create an imbalance in the body fast.

Sugar

Sugar is a surefire way to throw your body off balance. Recently, there has been a huge intake in how much we as a society consume sugar. Sugar seems to be sneaked into all kinds of products, even ones that aren't traditionally sweet like bread. In the USA, added sugars make up 17% of adults' calorie intake. It's no secret that sugar is bad, nor is it a new phenomenon to want to cut out sugar. However, with the highly addictive properties that sugar holds, letting go of your sweet addiction is harder than you may think. It's crucial, therefore, to examine some of the serious issues that sugar can cause to your body.

Diets high in sugar have been linked to diseases such as heart disease, which is the number one cause of all deaths worldwide. Aside from causing issues with your heart, sugar has also been connected to skin issues. You have probably come into contact with people who eat an unhealthy diet and have terrible skin as a result. Increased sugar consumption prompts your body to create more androgen secretion, oil production, and inflammation. This combination creates chaos under the surface of the skin and raises the risk of developing acne.

Eating a diet high in sugar also leads to obesity and resistance to insulin. This is a serious matter, putting you at high risk of developing type two diabetes. Obesity and insulin resistance are also serious risk factors for cancer. Beyond the aesthetic issues of weight gain, obesity can be a killer, and it's something that you should not take lightly.

Finally, sugar has also been proven to speed up the aging process and cause premature aging. A study by Leung et.al (2004) found that each 20-ounce daily serving of a sugar soda added 4.6 years of aging to someone.

These terrifying facts highlight the danger of sugar and how important it is to balance the amount of sugar that you are consuming.

Salt

Another imbalance-creator is salt. Before we examine the issues with salt, it's important to note that some salt is beneficial for health. Natural rock salt from the ocean and mountain salt such as pink Himalayan salt in moderate amounts are excellent for maintaining good health. However, the salt that you can buy at most stores and the salt that is added to your food is far more sinister.

Salt is composed of 40% sodium and 60% chloride, hence its scientific name, sodium chloride. Salt is excellent for both preserving foods and adding a little flavor to them. Good quality salt can have a host of benefits, including aiding muscle and nerve function and balancing the water and minerals in your body. The issues start to arise when too much salt is consumed. When salt is not eaten in moderation, it can begin to create problems that either cause immediate nuisances or long-term lingering damage.

Our bodies are designed to keep a strict ratio of sodium to water. Salt has the potential to upset this delicate balance, throwing the body off-kilter. When too much salt is consumed, you may feel a sense of bloating or puffiness as your body clings to water in your system to regulate the additional sodium. This bloating could present itself in the stomach, or even the hands, feet, and face. It even has the potential to make you weigh more on the scales than you would have before consuming the additional salt. Your kidneys lead this process, desperately trying to restore the balance of salt and water in your body.

After consuming too much salt in a meal, your body then begins to crave water. This can create an insatiable, intense thirst. If you don't comply with your body, you put yourself at risk of your sodium levels rising to a dangerous level. If this persists, a condition called hypernatremia can occur, where water leaks into the blood in a last-ditch attempt to dilute the unusual amount of sodium. This phenomenon can cause seizures, comas, and death if it is not treated.

Excess salt consumption has also been tied to a sharp rise in blood pressure. Salt creates a bigger blood volume flow throughout the bloodstream and arteries. This increased pumping of blood raises blood pressure, something that could be highly dangerous to those with predisposed heart conditions. This can be further amplified by those with obesity or a bad diet in general.

Worryingly, high salt diets have also been linked to stomach cancer (D'Elia et al., 2014). This is thought to happen as diets rich in salt put you at risk of developing inflammation of the stomach lining and stomach ulcers. Salt intake was also associated with a 68% higher risk of stomach cancer than those who ate moderate amounts of salt.

Seeing how easy it is to consume too much salt, it's crucial to try and regain proper balance when it comes to your salt consumption. Consider what foods you're eating that may have secret salt packed into them and watch how much additional salt you're adding to your meals. Where possible, swap out table salt for high-quality sea salt or mountain salt.

Acidic

You may have heard of the recent alkaline diet, which boasts some incredible health benefits. The opposite of this, therefore, is a diet rich in acidic foods. Acidic foods have been the subject of controversy for years, with many scientists recognizing that they are harmful to your health. By removing and limiting acidic foods from your diet, you're able to receive some of the benefits of the alkaline diet.

To determine whether a food is acidic or alkaline, the pH value needs to be measured. pH values range from zero to 14, with a neutral item such as water having a pH level of seven. Foods with a pH level under seven are classed as acidic, whereas foods scoring above seven are alkaline. Our blood is actually slightly alkaline, with a pH of 7.45 on average.

An alkaline diet, in general, is thought to be excellent for your health. As fruits and vegetables are alkaline by nature, consuming more of these has widespread advantages. This includes aiding bones, reducing muscle wastage, and helping to soothe the symptoms of chronic illnesses. Alkaline food also benefits the cardiovascular system and brain health, improving both memory and cognition. It also assists in the functioning of the enzyme system, so that vitamins like vitamin D and minerals like magnesium can be successfully absorbed.

Evidence also points to the damage that an acidic diet can cause. Scientists found that foods that have been metabolized leave behind a residue made up of chemicals that they call 'ash' (Fenton et al., 2008). When ash mixes with bodily fluids, it either forms an acid or alkali substance, which then causes a reaction in the body. When the ash is acidic, it begins to leach alkaline minerals like calcium from the bones, causing illnesses like osteoporosis.

Acidic foods such as meat, dairy, alcohol, soda, sweeteners, and table salt create mayhem in your system. On the other hand, alkaline foods are able to counteract the damage that eating acidic food does. Fruits and vegetables are the best sources of alkaline food. Even foods that we consider to be acidic, like lemons and limes, turn alkaline after they are metabolized. Further complications that can arise as a result of excess acid buildup include acid reflux, kidney problems, and acidosis, which is a buildup of acid in your tissue that is fatal if not treated. Trigger foods for these issues include fried, greasy foods, and full-fat dairy.

By incorporating less acidic and more alkaline foods into your diet, you can create a more alkaline pH level and reap all the rewards of doing so.

Spicy

Spicy food is a particular food group that seems to divide us all. Whether you're a lover of a spicy curry or hot sauce, or you tend to steer away from the spice, it's important to learn about what happens when we consume too much spicy food.

The reason why food tastes spicy is due to capsaicin, this raises the temperature of your tongue and burns any tissue that it encounters. Food that is extremely spicy even has the power to burn your skin, mucous membranes, and mouth (think hot chilies and peppers). For those who are not accustomed to eating hot food, the 'burning' sensation is even more prevalent.

Aside from the burn that spicy food can initially cause, there have also been strong links between spicy food and acid reflux. It also can cause gastroesophageal reflux disease, as the esophagus can become internally damaged. Further issues include heartburn and tooth erosion, as well as stomach issues as the capsaicin inflames the stomach lining.

Some even say that those who like spicy food aren't enjoying it for its particular flavor, but actually for the fact that it causes 'pain,' which some people enjoy. However, consuming too much spicy food can reduce taste and make it hard for spice-lovers to distinguish between flavors. The capsaicin numbs the tongue's pain sensors and even confuses signals in the brain related to taste. Prolonged consumption of extremely spicy food can cause irreversible damage to the taste buds.

Another interesting negative effect of having an imbalance of too much spicy food in your diet is that it can cause insomnia. A study on people who consume spicy food showed that they took longer to get to sleep and spent less time in deep sleep states (Edwards et al., 1992). This is connected to the capsaicin in the spicy food elevating the temperature of their bodies.

Although there are several issues with spicy food, it's also important to note that in moderation, it does have some excellent qualities. Hot food has the power to increase metabolism and blood circulation, and even to be good for your heart. However, the key, as with all of the other types of food explored in this chapter, is to consume them in a balanced manner.

When you can eat these items in moderation, ensuring that you are not throwing your body off balance, you take the first key step in creating holistic health.

Bitter

The final classification of food that can cause an imbalance in the body is bitter foods. Bitter foods can be described as anything with a strong unpleasant flavor that is neither salty nor sour. Vegetables, fruits, herbs, and plants can all be classed as bitter. Classic examples include brussels sprouts, cabbage, cocoa, coffee, wine, orange, and tea. A notable aftertaste can often be recognized after eating one of these foods.

In terms of their effect on your health, bitter foods actually contain very few helpful compounds and nutrients. They can often signal toxicity, with bitter foods aligning with acidity or negative chemical reactions. Negative reactions can occur after consuming a lot of bitter foods, including a loss of appetite, and upset stomachs in children.

One of the top antonyms for bitterness is artificial sweeteners. These sweeteners are commonly added to many of the food and drink items that are seen in stores today. With the huge surge in popularity of diet food and drinks and "low sugar" items, it seems that sweeteners are now even more popular than sugar. Don't be fooled by the calorie count on the pack though, sweeteners are bad news for your health. Side effects include an increase in appetite, weight gain, rewiring of brain chemistry, and a raised body temperature. Long-term effects even show that you're at risk of brain tumors, kidney stones, and diabetes with daily consumption of sweeteners.

Rather than trying to counteract bitter foods with sweeteners, select alternatives that you're happy to eat in their natural form. The key is to try and minimize all of the 'extra' things that you're adding to food, instead opting to eat them as they come.

Foods to Avoid

To get started right away, there are several foods that you can eliminate from your diet. Rather than thinking of losing something, see it as you're making more room in your diet to add in things that will be better for your health.

White Refined Sugar

First of all, begin by removing all white refined sugar from your diet. Sugar is one of the worst things that we can consume. This highly addictive substance has been added to so many of our food products, and sometimes it can be tempting to add sugar to food to satisfy your sweet tooth. When sugar is found in certain foods naturally, this is often okay, as it's usually in a moderate amount. However, society today consumes so much excess sugar that we need to be particularly suspicious of the food that we are eating.

Sugar has a detrimental effect on our weight, teeth, mood, and energy. You have most likely experienced what is known as a "sugar crash" when you feel exhausted after consuming a high sugar snack. This rollercoaster of rush and crash causes a strong addiction to sugar that may take weeks to shift. On average, it takes a person three to four weeks to completely detox from sugar. Some serious perseverance is needed to break free of the sugar cycle.

So why is sugar so addictive? Sugar releases dopamine into the brain, which creates the same effect as illegal drugs. Those choosing to eliminate sugar from their diet also experience withdrawal symptoms just like someone removing drugs from their life would. The cravings will be difficult at first, but the wonderful benefits of a sugar-free life surely outweigh this. To help you with the transition to a sugar-free life, consider incorporating naturally sweet foods such as fruits and dates.

White Refined Flour

What if you were to review all of the white refined food products that you currently eat? How many of the bread, pasta, and grains that you eat are white? Opting for the brown and whole-grain versions of foods will help to fill you up by providing slow-release energy, and stop the blood sugar spike that you get with white refined foods. Grabbing items like cakes and bread cause glucose spikes in your blood that can lead to dangerous issues such as diabetes.

The lack of fiber in these foods also hinders your digestion, opening you up to the risk of inflammation and infections. It's also a good idea to remove this from your diet for three to four weeks, just like sugar. You will most likely be able to see the benefits immediately.

Table Salt

We have examined some of the issues with salt earlier in this chapter. As you now know, refined table salt is something that should be immediately cut out of your diet. The problem with table salt is the extremely high mineral sodium content. When there is too much salt in the body, there is too much sodium, which attracts water. With excess water, you open yourself up to having too much fluid in your blood, creating high blood pressure. This high blood pressure can open you up to a range of issues such as hypertension, heart failure, and diabetes.

Table salt has also been stripped of all of the natural qualities that make it beneficial, such as its minerals. The processed table salt that is available to buy in stores also has a range of additives such as anti-caking ingredients, making it extremely toxic. Anti-caking agents contain aluminum, a carcinogenic substance that can also cause Alzheimer's disease. Remember to switch to natural salt, or to cut it out completely to avoid these frightening side effects.

Dairy

Dairy is one of the most genetically modified food groups that there is. As techniques are rolled out to increase the productivity of the meat, bioengineering hormone injections such as the bovine growth hormone aim to make cows larger than ever. The aim is to produce cows that have as much meat as possible, making them more profitable. These hormones are also used to increase milk production, giving the dairy corporations more bang for their buck.

Unfortunately, this not only has negative effects on the animal, but it has a knock-on effect on the humans consuming it too. The hormones create infections in the cow's udders such as mastitis. This then creates blood and pus which ends up straight in the milk that you drink. If you have to eat or drink dairy, try to seek it from local farms or organic markets.

Corn

One other highly genetically modified food is corn. About 88% of corn grown in the US is now genetically modified, with farmers in every state growing GMO corn. Products that use corn as an ingredient are also affected, such as chips or baked goods.

Soy

Soy is also highly genetically modified. Often considered a health food due to its prevalence in tofu and vegetarian food, soy has been genetically modified to be resistant to herbicides. Look out for soybean oil and soy flour as ingredients to ensure that you're steering clear of them.

Canola Oil

Canola oil is not only unhealthy, it is also one of the most genetically modified oils and has been since as early as 1996. Currently, around 90% of canola plants in the US are genetically modified, meaning that the chances of eating GMO canola are huge.

Papaya

Don't let the fact that it is a fruit fool you–papayas are significantly genetically modified. GMO papayas have been grown in Hawaii since 1999, with modifications designed to delay the fruit's maturity.

Meat

Meat should also be avoided where possible, in particular, chicken and beef. The animals are badly fed and pumped full of hormones and other chemicals that you will ultimately be ingesting. Unfortunately, the US is the leading producer of commercially-reared animals.

Aspartame

Finally, aspartame is something that you should be cutting out immediately. Aspartame is an additive sweetener that's super toxic. It is even created through the use of genetically modified bacteria. This sneaky sweetener is often added to diet soda drinks to fool you into thinking that they are healthy. It can cause headaches and nausea when consumed regularly.

I have been avoiding processed, GMO, and non-natural foods for over twenty-five years now. I am living proof that if I can do it, you can too. The first few weeks may be hard, but once you're past this, you'll begin to see the benefits that will have you hooked for a lifetime. As your body adjusts to the new, healthy food that you're consuming, you will begin to crave organic natural foods. These are the foods that your body was always meant to eat. After a while, the thought of eating processed, GMO foods will make you feel sick. Stay

strong and persistent on your transition and the results
will be astonishing.

Chapter 4:

The Third Imbalance Is People's Mindset and Condition

Your mind is such a powerful muscle, its condition can transform your physical health. Creating the optimum mindset is integral to holistic health. However, there are a plethora of risks in modern society that can cause your mindset and condition to become imbalanced. Learning about these and being able to protect yourself from as many as possible will place you in the best possible position to achieve holistic health. There are so many different ways in which you can become sick. Uncovering some of the different ways will mean that you can actively try not to engage in these activities or environments. While you may not be able to do this for all of the points, you can at least make a conscious effort to try to at least combat some.

Environment

Your environment plays a massive part in your holistic health journey. It doesn't take an expert to figure out that having a peaceful, sanitary, and relaxing environment will do wonders for your health. Not only does a clean and organized environment do amazing things for your mental health and productivity, but it also decreases the likelihood that you will be exposed to germs.

Unsanitary conditions don't just include slums and sewers, your home could be hiding a whole host of unsanitary items that appear to be clean. Educating yourself on areas that germs love to hide and multiply will help you to step up your cleaning routine and ultimately eliminate as many germs as possible. By doing this, you will help to protect yourself against becoming sick.

The first breeding ground for germs and illness is your bed. This may surprise you, but the average person sheds around half an ounce of dead skin every single week. These skin cells become trapped in your sheets, attracting bugs and parasites such as dust mites. These mites leave behind fecal matter that can cause skin irritations such as eczema and infections. They can also cause allergies to flare up, making you incredibly susceptible to sickness. Cleaning your bed sheets in hot water weekly will help to alleviate this.

Another culprit for germ-spreading in your home could be your heating or cooling system. When dust builds up in the pipes of these devices, it can end up forming mold, which is seriously detrimental to your health. Mold is particularly dangerous, as it can cause illnesses such as migraines, nausea, congestion, and asthma. In addition to this, other toxins can become trapped in the dust, making their way into your lungs as the air circulates. If there is only a small buildup in the pipes, cleaning them is appropriate, however, for very contaminated pipes, removal and replacement may be needed.

A further breeding ground for germs is your refrigerator. Even if at first glance it appears to be clean, invisible germs could be lurking on the surfaces and drawers. Organisms such as salmonella and E.coli that can cause stomach bugs and kidney failure are completely invisible to the naked eye. It's critical to clean your fridge carefully every month, including wiping down all of the shelves to avoid sickness.

Finally, even though they're meant to help to protect you from sickness, most household cleaning products are highly toxic. Loaded with dangerous chemicals and even carcinogens such as formaldehyde and perchloroethylene, you need to be extremely careful what cleaning products you let into your home. As science has advanced, there are lots of safe and natural cleaning products now available in stores. You may even want to opt for using a homemade mix of powerful cleaning ingredients like lemon, apple cider vinegar, and baking soda. This way you know that you're successfully keeping both sickness and toxins out of your home.

Socioeconomic Factors

Did you know that your socioeconomic standing, or how poor you are, directly affects your health? Sadly, being poor can harm many areas of your life, including your health. Evidence has pointed to the fact that living in poverty has the power to alter your gene expression. Exposure to poverty created children who had higher levels of stress hormones, higher blood pressure, and higher BMIs than children from more privileged backgrounds. This makes them more vulnerable to disease later in life.

Certain environmental factors can be tied to the link between poverty and health. For example, those who experience poverty are unlikely to be able to afford high-quality organic food or supplements. As convenience foods are far more cheaply priced than organic fruit and vegetables, they are the clear choice for those with a lack of funds. Exercise may also be difficult, with access to gyms or sporting equipment restricted by high costs. The anxiety of living in poverty is also a pivotal factor, with a study finding that living in poverty is a stronger predictor of mental health issues than going to war (Trani, & Bakhshi, 2013).

While you may not be able to do anything about the immediate circumstances that you live in, it's important to at least acknowledge the effect that they have.

High Stress

As we briefly touched on before, high levels of stress take a heavy toll on the immune system. This opens you up to be more susceptible to sickness and disease. High stress also does further mental and physical damage if it is not treated. As stress hormones rocket through your body, they create tension and inflammation that can ultimately damage your organs.

Further damage caused by stress includes chronic migraines, memory problems, high blood pressure, mental health conditions, fertility issues, and an increased risk of cancer. These frightening facts highlight how important it is to manage your stress correctly. To help treat this, identify what stressors in your life are triggers for you and try to limit them. You may also want to consider some relaxing exercises such as meditation, yoga, and breathing techniques.

Coping Mechanisms

Stress alone can be extremely detrimental to your health, but when you're able to utilize positive coping mechanisms, you harness the ability to bounce back. If you're unsure what a coping mechanism is—it's simply any strategy that you use to overcome a tough time. When faced with stress, we often adopt either positive or negative coping mechanisms to get through it. As you may have guessed, positive coping mechanisms are the ones that you should strive to use. These will have a positive effect on you and your physical and mental health. Negative mechanisms are often harmful and unhealthy but offer convenience and quick results, so they can be very tempting.

To start creating positive coping mechanisms that you can immediately integrate into your routine, try to start by confronting what is stressing you out. It may be a problem at work, a break-up, or even the stress of having an illness. Confronting what is stressing you out, whether it's addressing a person, problem, or your own emotions, will be an amazing first step toward inner peace. Other positive coping mechanisms include eating healthily, exercising, and channeling your stress into a hobby. Whatever you feel will help to alleviate your stress without causing you any harm is a wonderful way to rechannel stress.

Sometimes, you may get to the stage where you feel as if you are losing control over your life due to extreme stress. Using these positive coping techniques will help you to reestablish a routine and regain control once again. Do not fall into the trap of being a victim, instead, take ownership and step back into the driver's seat of your life.

Untreated Depression and Anxiety

Having untreated mental disorders such as anxiety and depression can make you more susceptible to a wide range of diseases, including cancer. There is a strong link between mental and physical health. People who suffer from mental disorders such as anxiety and depression have a higher risk of experiencing physical ailments.

The side-effects of mental illnesses can decrease energy levels and cognitive functioning, meaning that it's more difficult to adhere to healthy behaviors. Keeping a routine and staying motivated to keep on top of your health becomes a lot harder when you're suffering from a mental health problem. It may be more convenient to develop unhealthy sleeping and eating habits, which in turn negatively affect your immune system. As you now know, this then opens the door to a range of diseases and illnesses.

The symptoms of depression include a constant 'sad' mood, loss of interest in everyday activities, fatigue, difficult concentration, difficulty sleeping, and appetite changes. Someone who has depression may simply have this condition alone, or they may also have anxiety (or vice versa). Symptoms of anxiety include excessive worrying, nausea, muscle tension, difficulty sleeping, avoidant behavior, and regular panic attacks. If you believe that you may have a mental disorder, ensure that you seek prompt treatment to help you on your holistic health journey.

Sedentary Lifestyle

In recent years, humans have become far more sedentary than ever. With desk jobs, more tech, and fewer reasons to get up and leave the house, inactive lifestyles are becoming the norm. The downside to this is that it opens you up to an array of potential health problems. When you sit for extended periods, you lose bone density and muscle mass but gain fat. After neglecting physical activity for some time, you also become susceptible to heart disease, osteoporosis, and certain cancers such as colon and breast cancer. Remember to either get up and take regular breaks during extended periods of sitting, or to schedule sport and exercise into your daily routine.

Loneliness

Chronic loneliness has swept across modern society, with technological advancements making us feel more alone than ever. This loneliness can have a crippling effect on our lives. When there is a lack of social connection in your life, it can trigger the same primal alerts as physical hunger, thirst, and pain (Cacioppo & Patrick, 2009). So when you feel a pang of loneliness, it's akin to being deprived of food.

Loneliness is often triggered by something. It could be your environment, or even the television shows that you watch. Whatever the trigger may be, once you've recognized it, try to practice some self-love and self-compassion. How would you soothe a friend who is experiencing loneliness? Rather than beating yourself up, approach your own emotions with a warm and understanding nature. Avoid criticizing and berating yourself, instead choose healthy behaviors such as the coping mechanisms that we explored earlier, this will help you to avoid becoming sick.

Sudden Loss

One surefire way to throw off your body's natural balance is to go through trauma. Trauma is unavoidable in life. We will all at some point or another experience a sudden loss or tragedy. The effect that this can have on our bodies can be seriously detrimental. Losses such as the loss of a loved one, a job, a reversal of finances, or even finding yourself in a natural disaster event all constitute a serious state of loss. This then goes hand in hand with you getting sick as your body struggles to cope with the trauma. In addition to this, your physical health is often the last thing on your mind at times like this. This then causes your eating, sleeping, and exercise regimes to completely dissipate.

Whenever you receive the traumatic news of a loss, your body responds physically and can even start to shut down in order to process the trauma. You may experience this as an out-of-body experience, or a loss of control over your body. Symptoms of stress caused by a tragic loss include fatigue, change in appetite, nausea, trouble sleeping, and muscle aches. Over time, these can open the door to more serious illnesses. To help combat this, consider trying dance, music, massage, or reading books as healthy distractions.

Growing Old

Growing old is a risk for illness and disease as your body becomes more susceptible to ill health and infection. While nobody can stop the aging process, and growing old is a natural part of life, there are things that you can do to ensure that you remain healthy in your later years. You can begin living a healthy life immediately, giving you a better chance at good health as you grow old. You can start by looking after your eating habits, staying physically active, and reducing stress.

If you're currently older and looking for some low-impact ways to keep fit, water exercises, swimming, and cycling are great for fitness, and yoga and stretching work well for flexibility. You will also reap the benefits of healthy eating no matter what age you are, it is never too late to start.

Mindset

Mindset can also play a huge role in your physical condition. Incredibly, some people get sick because they expect to. Our mind is such a powerful tool that we can often unintentionally create disease by expecting it. Similarly, some people actually get sick, or even sicker after they are diagnosed with a disease. This expectation causes physical symptoms to manifest, or worsen. Your mindset can be used either to heal or harm you. It's up to you which route you want to take. Positive affirmations can be used to create a resilient mindset. These can either be gratitude-based and focus on feeling thankful for your good health, or healing-based, like stating that you're healing each and every day. Rather than giving up, a strong mindset will help you to find solutions and ways to achieve good health.

There is also a common belief that some people get sick because they simply want to give up on life. When you are constantly sending signals from your brain to your body that you're ready to give up, it ultimately will listen. On the other hand, some people have nothing better to do than get sick, so their body also complies.

How is your current mindset affecting your health? Do you speak about your health in positive terms? Do you expect health to be your natural state? If not, some work needs to be done to uncover why you have the mindset that you do. Start by swapping out the negative thoughts and statements that you tell yourself every day. Replace them with mantras and empowering affirmations instead. You have the power to shape your life through the statements that you tell yourself every day. Just as you feed your body with the right food, you must feed your mind with positivity. Get your mindset right, and your health will flourish.

Section 3:

Holistic Medicine and Herbal Benefits

In this section, you will be taken on a wonderful tour of all of the miraculous benefits that holistic medicine and herbal healing have. In the previous sections, you learned about the definitions and history of holistic medicine, and then many of the most common ways that you can become sick. This section will connect the two, presenting holistic medicine and herbal healing as the way to heal your body naturally. You'll acquire a critical analysis of both the advantages and disadvantages of holistic healing, allowing you to make an informed decision as to whether it feels right for you, as well as gaining knowledge on how to find the best possible information sources to support your decision. If you're itching to learn how herbal healing can transform your health, the next section will act as your new go-to.

Chapter 5:

The Incredible Benefits of

Herbal Healing

To really motivate yourself on your holistic healing journey, there is no better way than to examine the amazing benefits that herbal healing offers. Herbalism offers gentle, safe, and effective remedies that predate any modern medicine. These wonderful remedies have been used for generations, long before any of the prescriptions that we're given today. It's important to note that herbal medicine must only be used after a consultation with an expert herbalist.

Herbalism uses herbs and plants in a medicinal context to cure all kinds of ailments. This kind of holistic healing can be controversial, as many people are skeptical of the benefits that simple plants are able to provide. However, herbalism has been used universally to treat diseases for years, and herbal medicine is not a new treatment by any means. Herbal medicine uses leaves, seeds, roots, flowers, and even spices for medicinal purposes, harnessing the power of nature for healing. Different plants have their own selection of medicinal benefits, with different plants having the ability to cure different diseases.

There are countless benefits to using herbal medicine, one of the main ones being that they are safe and effective. This gentle form of healing is far less invasive than certain drugs and surgery. Herbal medicine also fills you with powerful life force energy, which makes for easy assimilation in your body. It has the power to activate your cells, cleanse your system and absorb quickly into your vital organs. Another huge benefit is that this form of medicine often doesn't have the nasty side effects that modern medicine does, such as sickness and migraines. This is largely dependent on your current health status and your history of drug or treatment usage. There are a range of different herbs and combinations that work for all kinds of illnesses, from your skin to your heart, and even your brain. This highlights how safe and effective herbal medicine is, and that it should be a priority for anyone looking for a highly effective, yet safe and gentle treatment.

One key point to note, however, is that many untrustworthy sources have begun to market 'natural' remedies and herbal medicine that are not truly authentic. It's always a good idea to do plenty of research and to consult a professional as opposed to falling for flashy marketing.

Many of the pharmaceutical drugs that are available in this day and age are simply there to mask symptoms and provide some comfort (so long as you keep taking the medicine). Herbal medicine instead allows you to uncover *why* you're experiencing this discomfort. Not only will this prevent the illness from continuing, but it will also speed up your recovery, allowing you to reach good health sooner.

Another massive benefit is that herbal medicines are much more affordable to produce, and for you, the consumer, to purchase. Prescription medicines can be extremely expensive, especially for chronic conditions that require ongoing treatment. Herbal medicines on the other hand are far cheaper to cultivate, as they are naturally found, as opposed to man-made. These naturally sourced medicines will save you a large amount of money in the long run, as low production costs equal low retail costs.

As you learn how to manage your condition with herbs, you'll gain valuable insight into how to self-heal, which will help you to live a healthier life overall. You'll not only discover how to treat your condition, but also how to prevent future illnesses from forming. What could a healthier life do for you? You could have fewer medical bills, less time off work, more energy, and more time to spend with your loved ones, doing things that you enjoy.

Herbal medicine also has the brilliant bonus of being able to boost the immune system. The potent minerals, vitamins, and goodness infused into the herbs work to strengthen the entire body. This will help you not only to combat your current illness, but to prevent any future ones from coming on. Your ability to fight infection and disease will be enhanced, protecting you from the inside out.

In recent years, somewhat of a movement has formed where people no longer want to be dictated to when it comes to their health. Frustrated by the lack of results from modern medicine, many people have begun to seek alternative routes. One of these, of course, is herbal medicine. This allows people to take control of their own health, empowering them to take back the reins. The amazing thing about incorporating herbalism into your life is that it allows you to educate yourself on what your body needs. As opposed to just treating symptoms when they appear, you will be able to identify the underlying problem and treat that condition. The knowledge that you will gain about yourself, your body, and your health, will be invaluable.

Self-empowerment is an extremely important skill to develop on your holistic healing journey. You may feel frustrated that you don't have control over your health but it's possible to completely eradicate this feeling with self-empowerment. Self-empowerment involves learning about yourself, understanding your inner power, and taking steps to take control of your health. The steps below will help you to utilize self-empowerment as a tool to supercharge your holistic healing process.

Responsibility

You may fall into the trap of believing that your health is totally out of your control. Especially with some of the more serious conditions, it can seem incredibly daunting and you may feel as if there is nothing that you can do. The first step to take in combating this is to take responsibility for your own health. Choosing to take responsibility for the results (or lack thereof) that you're experiencing will give you an immediate sense of control. Taking responsibility for your health is the single most important thing that you can do to empower yourself. Remember that in holistic healing, you need to consider your whole system and not just one organ or symptom. It is your responsibility to ensure that everything is working in unison and that you are not focusing on separate issues. This is *your* life, it's not anyone else's responsibility, nor should it be left to chance alone. Start to love yourself and treat your body with the respect and honor that it truly deserves.

Management

To truly empower yourself, an element of good management is needed. Developing your management skills and using them to help manage your condition will give you a true sense of control. Rather than allowing fate or the advice of a doctor alone to dictate how you manage your health, instead, step into the captain position. Learn how to manage your health well. This could include creating a schedule of when you need to take your herbal medicine, scheduling time for physical activity, or setting reminders to drink enough water each day. Learn to have some discipline when it comes to your health, and you'll surely see some great results.

Experience

Are you someone that gets stuck in their comfort zone? We as humans enjoy our creature comforts so much that it can sometimes be to our detriment. The fear of new experiences or trying new things has the potential to hold us back. Instead, seek out new experiences, as they may pave new paths to health. Try out different methods, experiment with new ideas, or even try to experience more in life. This is comparable to eating new, exciting food in an exotic foreign country. You may be skeptical at first, but after you try it, you wonder where this incredible food has been all your life! One amazing way to get started with this is to begin the transition over to natural organic food. As you learn about all of the wonderful recipes, combinations, and foods that you had never even heard of before, you're able to take your tastebuds on a journey of discovery.

Reliability

Many of us go through life simply accepting what we are told, without applying our critical thinking skills at all. There is nothing wrong with being inquisitive, and questioning whatever product, system, or service you are getting. This includes your health too. Begin to question the validity and reliability of the information that you're consuming. Check multiple sources, look at contrasting views, and use your masterful critiques to discern whether a piece of information sits right with you or not. With the internet, it's easy to fall victim to fake news and opinion cloaked as fact, so make sure that your research is always thorough.

You now have a solid insight into how herbal healing can benefit not only your health but your overall life too. In true holistic form, it's significant to look at how herbal medicine can improve your bank balance, quality of life, and even your happiness, as well as just your health. When you combine the known advantages of herbal medicine with the powerful self-empowerment techniques outlined in this chapter, you have a killer combination for all kinds of diseases and illnesses.

Chapter 6:

The Advantages vs Disadvantages of Holistic Herbal Medicine

As with any idea or philosophy, it's important to critically weigh up both the advantages and disadvantages so that you can make an informed decision as to whether it's for you or not. As the landscape of medicine changes, with holistic and herbal treatments gaining vast popularity, there will of course always be some disadvantages to weigh up too.

While holistic medicine is often met with a cold reception from the scientific community, it has a long history of success, spanning decades. There are some noteworthy advantages that should factor into your decision as to whether to adopt a holistic approach to your healing.

Empowerment

As we touched on in the previous chapter, one of the wonderful benefits of herbal medicine is that it offers an element of empowerment. With modern medicine taking away your control and having you dictated to by medical professionals, you can often feel disheartened. You have to live by the rules and recommendations of a doctor who may not know what's best for you and your own body's makeup. With holistic healing, you're able to understand the power that you hold. Your body has an innate ability to heal. Think about when you cut your finger, your body magically heals the cut and after some time it's as if it never happened. When you're able to connect with the powerful healing energy that your body already has, you can utilize it to heal your conditions the natural way.

Rather than taking medicine to stifle symptoms, you can educate yourself on a healthy lifestyle and make the necessary changes needed to elevate your health. This includes self-care, learning how to fuel your body with the correct nutrition, and what herbal remedies will assist your treatment. Having more control over your health will fill you with confidence and empower you to reach optimum health.

A Natural Alternative

Chemicals have found their way into pretty much everything in our lives. From the air that we breathe to the water that we drink, and especially in modern medicine. The buildup of these chemicals can cause countless issues, so looking to herbal medicine that uses natural healing power instead is a great alternative. There is also no rule to say that you can't use a combination of both pharmaceutical and holistic products. Holistic healing can offer a welcome release from the harsh effects of pharmaceutical drugs. This may help you to cut down on the number of pharmaceutical products that you're using, or even eradicate them from your treatment regime.

The perks of herbal medicine are that it uses the body's natural healing processes for treatment. The way that it can happen all comes down to the ingredients that are found in herbal medicine. They can often be traced back to vitamins and minerals that are found in the body. Making use of these naturally occurring ingredients is a safer and more gentle alternative to harsh, toxic chemicals that are found in modern medicine.

Cost-Effective

A huge benefit of holistic healing treatments is that they can often provide a far more cost-effective solution to modern medicine and pharmaceutical drugs. It's common knowledge that pharmaceutical drugs can cost hundreds of dollars. If you suffer from a chronic, long-term condition, or you have multiple illnesses, this can become extremely expensive. Holistic remedies offer a less expensive treatment route. From therapies such as acupuncture, massage, and cupping, to natural herbal remedies and dietary supplements, holistic treatments are significantly cheaper than drugs and surgery. As herbs are naturally occurring, they don't come with many of the additional costs that modern medical drugs do. On top of the production of the treatment itself, pharmaceutical drugs have extra overheads such as research, testing, and marketing fees.

As you're embarking on your healing journey, treatments are always likely to be more effective if you're able to keep your stress levels down. Having money troubles and worrying about where the money for your next medical bill is going to come from is only going to add to your sense of stress. Therefore, choosing the most cost-effective treatment route makes sense to calm your mind and allow you to stay in a positive, healing energy state.

Multi-Tasking

While modern medicine centers on finding a symptom and providing relief for that one particular symptom, holistic medicine takes an entirely different approach. Holistic treatments can heal and protect against a variety of illnesses and symptoms simultaneously. Rather than just treating a skin, heart, or mental condition, holistic and herbal medicine will improve your health as a whole. The "side-effects" of holistic healing are positive in this case, with holistic remedies able to treat the conditions below as a bonus:

- Cancer
- Stroke
- Skin disease (e.g eczema, acne, psoriasis)
- Heart disease

- High blood pressure
- Anxiety and depression
- Fatigue
- Chronic pain

This all ties in with the basis of holistic medical principles. When you view the body as a whole and ensure that health is viewed in a holistic manner, overall optimum health is the outcome. You will most likely find that throughout your holistic treatment process you will experience effects such as increased energy, improved skin, and enhanced cognitive skills. As you learned previously in this book, we are not the sum of our individual parts, but the sum of all parts working together.

Herbal medicine is also a fantastic alternative to conditions that aren't responding well to modern medicine. Chronic conditions can often see a plateau after long-term use of pharmaceutical medicine. Holistic treatments can help here—with herbal medicines providing more effective treatment for long-term conditions.

Treating the Whole Person

What sets apart holistic healing from modern medicine is the emphasis on you as a person. Often, doctors will remove the cause of an illness, disregarding factors such as your emotional, mental, and spiritual well-being. These elements are overlooked, with emphasis placed only on the visible symptoms. Sometimes illness has causes that require further investigation and understanding. By ensuring that mind, body, and spirit are all working cohesively, you're realizing that your illness is not a distinct entity from you.

Whole-body care is particularly important when aiming for optimum health. Imagine your local hospital—you'll probably be able to visualize all of the different departments and the doctors with specializations in their individual areas. This fragmentation of modern medicine emphasizes a focus on just one particular body part. There is a doctor or specialist for every single body part and even for many individual diseases. This separated approach means that it's highly rare that a doctor will take into account your emotional, mental, or spiritual well-being. Your illness may be able to be traced back to an emotional imbalance, a trauma, or a behavior that you need to work on. Holistic medicine and alternative remedies take all of this into account.

As a result of this, a greater amount of personal attention is placed on you as the patient. Alternative medical practitioners are able to create detailed plans, with more attention placed on all areas of your well-being. This is a stark contrast to the time-poor, overbooked traditional doctors.

Less Side-Effects

As we explored previously, the "side-effects" of holistic medicine are actually rather positive. On the other hand, the side effects of pharmaceutical medicine can be the total opposite. From adverse or allergic reactions to uncomfortable day-to-day hindrances such as headaches and nausea, the side effects of modern medical treatments can be difficult to live with. If you've ever taken prescription medicine, you may have noticed the extensive side-effects list on the treatment pamphlet. The scary truth is that beyond the effects listed, there are often many more that the pharma companies are unaware of yet.

In comparison, the majority of herbal medicines are tolerated well by most patients. There have been noticeably fewer reports of adverse effects from holistic and herbal treatments. Even after years of treatment, herbal treatments have proved to be safe for continued usage.

No Prescription Required

A big advantage of holistic remedies is that you're able to access treatment without the waiting time or inconvenience of having to have a prescription filled. It can be troublesome to have to consult a doctor every single time you need to get some medicine. The ease of being able to walk into a store and purchase herbal medicine makes it far more accessible than pharmaceutical drugs. The widespread availability of herbal medicines in stores can also be both time and money-saving.

You may even want to consider growing your own herbs for medicinal purposes. Cultivating a mini-garden full of herbs and holistic plants will give you on-demand access to treatment at your fingertips. Herbs such as chamomile and peppermint are simple to grow and easy to look after. This is also a sustainable alternative that's kind to the planet.

While there are countless wonderful advantages to holistic medicine, it's equally important to examine some of the disadvantages. There has been somewhat of a resistance to holistic healing, with many critics raising concern over its effectiveness. Below are some of the key arguments against holistic healing, so that you can fairly weigh up whether it is right for you.

Not for Serious Illnesses

While herbal medicines are effective at treating a number of conditions, they are unable to treat many serious illnesses. Some ailments do require surgery or more complex treatment options. For example, broken bones or a heart attack will need more than herbal medication to heal. Many trauma-based injuries need more sophisticated care far beyond what herbal remedies can offer.

Trial and Error Nature

In some cases, especially where individuals undertake holistic medical treatments without professional consultation, a "trial and error" scenario is created. You may find that when embarking on your personal holistic healing journey that not having a prescription can actually be confusing. There is a lack of close monitoring of your health and reaction to holistic medicine unless you are working with a practitioner. You may start a course of one particular herb, not realizing that your condition is caused by something that would require an alternative herb.

There is also less of a clear-cut treatment prognosis with holistic medicine. While modern medicine offers guidelines and expectations to patients, such as the promise that pills will heal an infection in two weeks, holistic medicine is unable to do so. As you as a patient are totally unique in the eyes of the holistic community, your treatment time may be entirely different from someone else. In general, the curing period when using herbal medicine is also remarkably longer in comparison to modern medicine.

Lack of Approval and Research

Perhaps the most famous of all the arguments against holistic medicine, the lack of government and scientific research is an important factor to consider. The government does not (and has never) approved of any form of holistic or herbal medicine. It even goes as far as to warn people about the use of herbal medicine, advising people that they are to take it at their own risk. Even after mass public outcry into the need to fund research studies on holistic medicine, evidence is very finite. Even as a couple of scientific studies begin to trickle through into the mainstream, there is a huge gap between research on modern and holistic medicine.

The issue with this lack of research is that it can grow the amount of subpar herbal treatments that are available on the market. For example, there have been instances of the wrong species of plant, accidental contamination with toxic substances, and incorrect dosage advice in herbal medicines that have been attributed to adverse effects. Herbal medicines can also cause allergic reactions if you are allergic to a particular herb without realizing that you are. The lack of proper education on holistic medicines perpetuates these issues, which could make the use of herbal treatments dangerous.

The lack of research and knowledge into holistic medicines also means that there is a risk that they can interact with prescription medication. In scientific research, rigorous testing is done to ensure that any reactions between medicines are listed alongside the medicine. Traditional doctors will also usually check when prescribing medication that the patient is not taking any medication that could react badly with the new meds. Even though holistic remedies are natural, they still have the potential to create an adverse reaction. This can even happen in conjunction with over-the-counter medicines too.

Unethical Marketing

In recent years, herbal medicine has gained somewhat of a link to unethical marketing practices. This promotes the stereotype that herbal medicine is a 'scam,' or a 'fad.' Not all health products that are marketed today are genuine holistic treatments. Many dietary supplements and holistic remedies are simply gimmicks masquerading as natural remedies. These types of unethical products can often be spotted by the unrealistic claims that they make. Any products that have excessive marketing that promote miracle cures, overnight results, or top-secret ingredients are likely to be ineffective. Marketers use the umbrella of natural products to try and sell inefficient items that are not actually beneficial to your health.

As you've now seen, there are several advantages and disadvantages to using holistic herbal medicine. This is not a decision that should be taken lightly. You may wish to continue your research and look into this in-depth, but ultimately the decision as to whether to transition into herbal healing is completely up to you. As with anything, evaluation is key to help you make the decision that is right for you. Your intuition and gut will also play a huge role in your decision. Trust that with correct research and your strong intuition, that you will make the right choice. Your health is in your control, as long as you're willing to put yourself in the driver's seat.

Chapter 7:

Identifying Good Quality

Sources of Information

With all of the conflicting information out there, it can be extremely hard to distinguish what information is genuine. Many companies use clever marketing techniques to throw you off, and some companies don't display their ingredients altogether. When you're researching online about the information on holistic healing, there are so many sources that it can be overwhelming, and sources can often have clashing standpoints.

One way to ascertain whether a holistic treatment or medicine is right for you is to look at product reviews. Reviews from real people just like you who are trying to heal naturally will provide an insight into what the treatment is really like. This is where people are most likely to report whether there were any issues, side effects, or adverse reactions. They may also talk you through the benefits, what to expect, and document some of their results. While reviews are an excellent way to gather information on holistic treatments, there are a few points that you should keep an eye out for. Seen frequently with marketed products (as opposed to just plants or herbs), fake reviews are rife in the online space. Companies have been known to pay or bribe people to provide a good review in exchange for something. Some of the lazier companies even use bots or paid-for services to flood sites with positive reviews. Always look carefully at the profiles or accounts in the review section. Do the reviews all sound very similar? Has the reviewer only ever left one review before according to their profile? These are telltale signs that a review is ingenuine.

While product reviews are great for evaluating commercial products, herbal supplements are not put under the microscope to the same degree as this. Herbal treatments tend to not be under the same scrutiny and regulation as medications. However, do not let this fool you. Herbs and herbal products can create strong effects on your body. Even though they are labeled as 'natural,' they should be consumed with caution. Before you embark on your holistic treatment regime, it's ideal to do some research before you invest. Aside from the benefits, look for its interaction with other mediation, side effects, and any potential warnings. This is particularly important if you have a long-term chronic health condition, you're pregnant, or you breastfeed.

There are some regulations in place to control the supply of herbal supplements and medicines, but they are nowhere near as stringent as the measures in place for over-the-counter medicine. In the US, the Food and Drug Administration department (FDA) regulates the holistic medicine products industry. Herbal supplements come under the umbrella of "dietary supplements," meaning that despite the context in which they are taken, they don't need the official FDA stamp of approval to be sold. There are some regulations on holistic products, one being that supplements have to be correctly labeled and free from contaminants. All holistic supplements also need some research behind them to indicate that they are beneficial to health, but the FDA has not evaluated the claim. The FDA also has the right to take action against any companies who make false and unsubstantiated medical claims. This provides somewhat of a level of reassurance that the supplements available on the market are quality and that any dangerous ones are withdrawn from the market.

While this offers a layer of protection, there is no guarantee that holistic medicine is safe to use for everyone. Of course, just like any medicine, there will always be certain groups who should not use it at all. The active ingredients that make herbal medicine so magically effective for some will be the exact reason why others have an adverse reaction. These potent and powerful ingredients can become harmful when they interact with prescription drugs. If you're taking medication currently, it's crucial to speak with your doctor to understand if you're able to mix the two safely. Some over-the-counter medications such as aspirin and blood pressure medications can also interfere with holistic treatments, so if in doubt, consult a professional. Herbal medicine also has the potential to stop anesthesia from being effective, so it's wise to not take it when having surgery.

If you're wondering what is in a supplement that you're considering taking, a great place to start your investigation is on the product label. The FDA requires all supplement labels to include information on the name and address of the manufacturer, a full list of ingredients, and the recommended serving size. If you're ever unsure about an ingredient or item on the label, you can research it online or ask a holistic practitioner for advice. Another excellent source is the Dietary Supplement Label Database. This helpful tool is found on the US National Institute of Health website and allows you to research products by name, uses, active ingredients, and manufacturer.

You may have seen some eye-catching claims made by manufacturers of holistic supplements and remedies. While these manufacturers are responsible for ensuring that claims aren't false or misleading, they are not required to submit evidence of this to the FDA. This means that you often need to do your own research to decipher whether a product is truly effective, or just has persuasive marketing. To help you to evaluate this, there are a number of reputable sources online that you can use to do some in-depth research, The National Center for Complementary and Integrative Health and the Office of Dietary Supplements have plenty of information to help you make an informed decision as to whether a treatment is right for you. Consulting your holistic doctor or practitioner is always a great idea too, as they will often be able to raise any concerns with you immediately. If you're still in doubt, you can always contact the manufacturer of a product directly to ask direct questions about evidence that they have to back up their health claims.

Aside from your medication and supplements, your food also requires some research to ensure that you're putting the best possible fuel into your body. In Chapter four, you learned about the importance of putting high-quality food into your body. Learning more about the effect of what you eat on your body can help to complement the work of the holistic medicine that you take. When you're looking into the food that you eat, it's best to start with the farm that it's produced on. As you try to incorporate more organic, healthy whole foods into your diet, you should be aiming to purchase food that you can trace back to a particular farm or manufacturer. If you can shop locally on farms that you're able to visit in person, this is ideal, however, many people, unfortunately, do not have the option to do so.

Another factor to take into consideration is the transportation of your food. Learning how far your food had to travel to reach you will give you an indication of its quality. Try to find out what city or country your food is labeled as coming from. This is important as food products can begin to deteriorate or become contaminated by microorganisms during the transportation stages in the logistics chain. Before food reaches your plate, it often has to go through a long journey to get there. Issues including too high of a temperature and too much humidity can result in food spoilage. Ensuring that your food has traveled in temperature-controlled transportation will minimize any risks. You may also wish to discover whether your food options have traveled by road, train, sea, or air, as the longer that the food takes to get to you, the higher the risk of contamination is.

When you're adding more organic food into your diet, you may also want to look into whether your 'organic' food is legitimate. Certifications such as the USDA organic label are excellent ways to ensure that you are eating genuine organic produce. The USDA label is formulated with a certification system that verifies all farmers and producers all across the world. There are five steps for a farmer to become accredited with a USDA label.

1. **Develop a plan:** Farmers have to create an organic system plan to explain how they will comply with the USDA regulations. Plans will cover everything from fertilizing, harvesting, storing, and transporting, as well as a list of all substances used throughout.

2. **Implement the plan:** The farmer will then carry out their plan with a certified agent ensuring that all of the organic produce meets the USDA standards.

3. **Inspection:** Agents will inspect and carry out top-to-bottom checks across the entire farm or facility. This includes all soil, crops, livestock, and admin checks.

4. **Review:** The report will be reviewed and any potential risks assessed.

5. **Decision made:** A decision will finally be made as to whether the farm or facility meets all of the strict criteria to receive the certification.

As you can see, the rigorous checks that go into checking the safety and validity of organic produce through the USDA certification make it a highly trustworthy way of verifying that your organic food is safe. A final point regarding your food that you may want to look into is whether it is genetically modified. Genetic modification can have detrimental effects on your health, so looking up whether the food you eat is GMO or not will help to keep you as healthy as possible. For a good to be called as Non-GMO, it must be evaluated and passed as being compliant. There are four risk levels that GMO products are categorized into by the Non-GMO project (an excellent online source).

Risk	Definition	Examples
High Risk	Known to be genetically modified.	Canola, corn, papaya, soy, yellow summer squash, meat.
Low Risk	Not presently known to be genetically modified.	Avocados, lentils, tomatoes, spinach.
Non Risk	Not derived from biological organisms, so not eligible to be genetically modified.	N/A
Monitored Risk	Not presently known to be genetically modified, but are likely to be, or have been contaminated.	Apple, flax, mushroom, orange, pineapple, wheat.

While you may not be able to track down the origins of all of the food that you eat, looking at each stage of its journey onto your plate will help you to identify helpful information. If in doubt, contact the company that you bought the produce from. They should be open with you and let you know where your food has come from so that you can better understand its consequences on your health.

Sometimes, the best source of information can be to just strike up a conversation with real-life people. Visit holistic shops or areas where you think like minded people would hang out and start conversations about holistic healing. You may find people who have similar conditions to you, or who just have general tips on staying healthy holistically. If you're not able to do this, a great alternative could be to visit online message boards or communities. Look at results that are backed with data, or detailed testimonials to learn whether a particular treatment or herb is right for you. This also gives you the opportunity to message the poster and ask them specific questions to help you on your own journey.

If you feel satisfied after research that you're happy to try a product, it's a good idea to do so in a controlled and measured manner. Test the product each day in small increments, keeping a detailed record of how you feel and any reactions that you have. Make sure that you're not mixing it with any pharmaceutical or over-the-counter drugs that could have an adverse reaction. If in doubt, remember you can always consult a holistic doctor. It's better to be safe than sorry when it comes to anything that you ingest.

Results won't be immediate with holistic healing. From my own experience, I've noticed that most people begin to see some small results trickle in after around two weeks. For others, this initial healing can only show itself after around three to four weeks. If you're pleased with the result after four weeks, it's safe to continue using to rebalance your health. You're welcome to continue usage, or to stop using it when you feel that your body has regained balance. My suggestion would be to lower the dosage and take what is classed as a "maintenance dose." This will act like a health insurance for your body, ensuring that you have strong immunity defenses to fight off any illnesses. Of course, you should always consult your doctor to ensure that whatever you're going to take won't interfere with any pharmaceutical meds that you're taking.

Finding information can seem formidable at first, but don't be put off. Taking some time to do some proper research into what exactly you're putting into your body will give you true peace of mind. Ensure that you're always looking at good quality, unbiased sources and you'll be well on your way to a wealth of knowledge on holistic health.

Chapter 8:

Options for Herbal

Medicine Methods

Herbal medicine is an extremely broad term. With so many different methods of using herbs to heal the body, you may feel a little confused as to where to start. You also may have little to no understanding as to what is even out there in the herbal medicine space. Do not panic–everyone has to start somewhere. This chapter will help you to acquire all the knowledge that you need on the most popular herbal medicine methods. There are many ways to get the power of herbal medicine into your system. The route that you go down will largely be down to your personal preference.

Water

Water has long been linked to its incredible healing properties. With 80% of our body being made up of water, it's no wonder that this magical element is tied so closely to holistic healing. You can utilize the power of water to carry your herbal medicine into your body gently and safely. There are many different ways of using water for holistic healing.

Holistic Herbal Healing Teas (Organic)

A classic water-based method is to brew herbal tea. Herbal teas can have excellent therapeutic properties, with the added bonus that many are delicious to drink too! Herbal teas have antioxidant properties and are often naturally packed full of vitamins and minerals. As well as addressing your targeted problem, herbal teas can support your digestive and brain health, and boost your brain by aiding cognitive function.

By researching what herbs are best for your condition, you can identify which ones would work well to include in a herbal tea. You can either purchase them in a dried or powder format or use fresh ingredients and boil or simmer them in hot water to make a holistic healing tea. A similar style can be used to create all kinds of healing teas. Start with one tablespoon of your active ingredient (for example, ginger, turmeric, or peppermint), then add one cup of boiling water. Remove the mixture from the heat and allow it to simmer for around 15 minutes. If you don't like the taste of your main ingredient, you could try adding in some lemon, raw honey, or stevia to sweeten the taste. However, you will most likely find that after regular consumption, you'll learn to love the taste!

As with any herbal medicine, you should keep a close eye on any side effects that may occur. If you notice discomfort in your throat or an upset stomach, it's best to stop drinking the tea immediately.

Holistic Herbal Infusions (Organic)

As herbs are packed full of healing goodness, an ideal way to consume them is through herbal infusions. These ensure that you're consuming all of the oils and flavors from the herbs, allowing their healing properties to effectively enter your system. Infusions are made by soaking herbs in water until the herb's oils have been totally absorbed. You then drink the liquid to benefit from all of its holistic medicinal qualities. While tea only uses the leaves and flowers of the plant, infusions incorporate the roots and shoots too.

You will feel as if you're deeply connected to nature when drinking an infusion. Other herbal healing methods, such as taking pills or tablets, often don't have the same natural feel. They can also taste delicious, especially when you're a fan of the particular healing herb that you're using. You can consume herbal infusions cold or hot, either enjoyed over ice or in the style of a hot tea based on your personal preference.

Many herbs are suitable for use in your herbal infusion, however, tried and trusted ones include aloe vera, mint, thyme, camomile, sage, lavender, and nettle. Great tasting additions include ginger and any form of mint. Make sure that you look into which herbs you're mixing, as some may lead to a bad reaction when mixed. If you're unsure, consult a holistic doctor or look online for research or warnings.

To create your own holistic herbal infusion, place your chosen herbs into a glass container and pour boiling water over them until they are completely covered. Seal the jar to avoid the steam from escaping and allow the infusion to steep for around eight hours. Once they've steeped, strain the spent herbs from the water using a strainer and enjoy your infusion!

Holistic Herbal Decoctions (Organic)

Decoctions are a helpful alternative to infusions and are used when dealing with tough roots, or herbs that don't contain a lot of oil. If you've experimented with the previous two methods when trying to consume the best herb to treat your condition, but you're struggling to extract enough out of it, decoctions are ideal. They create a highly concentrated remedy that you can take just a teaspoon of for supercharged results. Decoctions are made by boiling either dried or fresh herbs in water. Doing so extracts all of their water-soluble goodness and works excellently for anyone who doesn't like to drink teas or infusions.

To make a herbal decoction, cut or ground your herbs so that it's easier to extract their healing properties. If you're dealing with a particularly stubborn, tough root, soak it in water for 12 hours before making your decoction. When you're ready, simply boil the herbs in distilled or spring water until around 50% of the water has evaporated. Remove it from the heat and strain it using a filter to create the finished product. One small point to note is that metal pots may react with certain astringent herbs and alter their taste, so opt for glass or porcelain containers where you can. Take a teaspoon of your decoction orally, or use it topically on an affected area for incredible results.

Holistic Herbal Tinctures (Organic)

Tinctures are liquid herbal extracts that are taken orally under the tongue, as this is the fastest way to get the herbs into your bloodstream. Typically, tinctures are extracted in alcohol, however, you can also use vegetable glycerine or apple cider vinegar. I would recommend apple cider vinegar, as it's natural, healthy, and can also be used for a variety of other things (like salad dressings). As tinctures are taken under the tongue, the body can rapidly make use of the herb's healing properties. The effect takes place much faster than the likes of tablets.

A huge plus when using tinctures is that they're very convenient and portable. As opposed to teas that would require an element of preparation, tinctures can be used anywhere on the go. Tinctures are taken through a small dropper bottle. Herbs are inserted into the bottle alongside the apple cider vinegar, and then a few drops are applied under the tongue. Typically, a standard adult dosage is two drops, two to three times a day. If you really dislike the taste of the tincture, you can always add a few drops into a glass of water and sweeten it with some honey.

Holistic Herbal Syrups (Organic)

If you have a sweet tooth, a herbal syrup could be the perfect way for you to ingest your holistic herbal goodness. A herbal syrup is made using a decoction, exactly like we explored in the previous paragraph. The decoction is simply mixed with sugar or honey. This not only makes it taste delicious but preserves the shelf life and creates a soothing application. Extra effects of this include soothing a sore throat, cough, or any digestive issues.

To create your herbal syrup, mix two parts of herbal decoction with one part of sugar or honey to create a 2:1 ratio. This syrup will preserve nicely, so feel free to store it in your favorite glass jar. You may even want to experiment with the ratio and find out how much sugar works for you. Some will prefer a slightly sweeter taste. The beauty of creating your own syrup is that you can personalize it to your liking.

Liquid

Holistic Herbal Infused Oils (Organic)

A herbal infused oil is an oil infused with the holistic power of the leaves, stems, roots, and flowers of a herb. The oil is made by allowing the natural materials to infuse into the oil for around four to six weeks in the sun. The oil allows for a double dose of benefits as it infuses with all the nourishment of the herbs.

To make your herbal infused oil, you'll first need to select a carrier oil. Most herbal constituents are too harsh to apply directly to your skin or consume, so they need a base oil to dilute them safely. Some excellent oils for this include olive, coconut, jojoba, or hemp oil. I would recommend using dried herbs for your oil infusion, as fresh herbs can often turn the oil rancid.

Holistic Herbal Essential Oils (Organic)

An alternative to infused oils is herbal essential oils. These are highly concentrated, potent oils, as opposed to infused oils, which are diluted with a carrier oil. They are so strong that the recommendation is never to apply them directly to the skin. Even consuming them in your mouth could cause burning. These should also be diluted in a carrier oil before use. To make the most of these potent oils, mix with a little bit of coconut or avocado oil and either place under your tongue, or apply topically.

Solid

Holistic Herbal Poultices (Organic)

As opposed to all of the other items in this chapter that you have to consume internally, poultices offer a topical application of herbs. The herb will still be absorbed directly into the bloodstream, but instead of consuming it, you apply it to the skin. They are also handy for use in first-aid contexts, such as on burns, cuts, bruises, or even sunburns. With a holistic herbal poultice, herbs are mixed with water or oil to create a paste that is spread onto the skin.

To create your herbal poultice, take your herb or selection of herbs and combine them with a little hot water so that they begin to moisten. Keep adding small amounts of water until the mixture forms a paste. You can then spread the paste over your desired area to allow it to absorb into your skin and enter your bloodstream.

Holistic Herbal Ointments and Salves (Organic)

Holistic herbal ointments encompass dried herbs into a mixture with fats or oils. As these contain no water, they form a separate layer on top of the skin that can carry the holistic medicinal constituents to the affected area. They are also excellent for drawing toxins out of a particular area. You can use herbal ointments or salves on a variety of conditions to soothe them too, such as burns, scrapes, bites, cuts, and bruises.

To create your holistic herbal ointment, melt beeswax into a large glass bowl that's set over a pan of boiling water. Chop and add fresh herbs, or throw in some dried herbs and simmer the mixture for fifteen minutes, ensuring that you're stirring regularly. Attach a jelly bag to the rim of a large jug with some string and pour in the liquid mixture, allowing it to filter through. Try to get as much of the hot herb mix through as possible. You may wish to wear some rubber gloves for this, as it can get messy! Pour the molten mixture into jars before it sets and seal when cooled.

Holistic Herbal Compresses (Organic)

Another excellent topical use for your holistic herbal medicine is to prepare a compress. You may have seen these before under a different name, as holistic practitioners call them everything from pouches, palls, or stems. They are used either to glide across the body or in conjunction with massage. Herbal compresses are great for soothing inflammation or pain, as well as getting the healing properties of the herb into your system via your skin.

You're also able to access additional benefits such as stress relief, muscle soothing, improved circulation, and stimulation of your internal organs. You can either heat the mixture and create a hot compress, or cool it in the fridge to soothe injury or inflammation. Simply select your herbs and wrap them into a compress. Steam the compress and then sweep it over your skin in a circular motion, using rolling movements and ensuring that you're pressing it into the skin as you move.

Powders, Pills, Capsules, and Vitamins (Organic)

Perhaps one of the most well-known ways to take your holistic herbal medicine, powders, pills, capsules, and vitamins are always a convenient choice. You may have seen examples of natural supplements such as probiotics, fatty acids, and vitamin and mineral tablets. Many of these are simply used to supplement nutritional deficiencies in your diet, but there are also numerous herbs and holistic treatments available in this form.

There are holistic treatments available in pill and powder format for a range of specific health needs. From improving the condition of your skin and nails to aiding gut and digestive function, and boosting your immune system, you're able to access vast benefits through their usage. In today's day and age where so much of our food is processed or susceptible to genetic modification, it's helpful to have easy ways to get more goodness into our bodies. Taking some natural supplements alongside a healthy diet will help to combat any imbalance.

When you're taking herbal medicine in the form of powders, pills, capsules, and vitamins, ensure that you're always doing your research. Look at how much of the active ingredient is present in the pill, as some manufacturers like to mix it with many other ingredients for an "all-in-one" solution. However, make sure that the dose you're taking is enough for you to get the results that you desire. As always, if you're in doubt, consult your holistic practitioner.

It's also important to ensure that you're opting for natural as opposed to synthetic vitamins. There is a big difference between the two, with synthetic supplements having a range of serious faults. Synthetic supplements are often packed with preservatives that allow them to last on shelves and in stockrooms for months or even years. The process that is used to create them is also vastly different from natural products. The finished product is usually a compound and not something that is naturally occurring. Synthetic supplements are not as bioavailable, absorbable, and therefore usable as proper vitamins are to your body. Rather than complete nutrients, they are simulated nutrients. Your body needs to recognize the whole, not just the individual compounds that make up an essential vitamin. Some can even be so artificial that your kidney will treat them as toxins.

To help you to distinguish synthetic supplements from natural ones, avoid supplements that use any words ending in '-ide,' '-acid,' or '-ate.' Also, avoid supplements that have 'dl' before their name.

However you decide to take your holistic herbal medicine, always ensure that you're properly researching your choice or consulting a holistic practitioner. You may wish to use a combination of methods, or you could find one that works perfectly for your condition. Experiment with the different methods and find what works best for your budget and lifestyle.

Section 4:

Take Action

In this section, you will receive all of the tools and tips that you need to take action and begin your holistic healing journey. You now have all of the knowledge that you need to make changes and take initiative for your own health. The chapters that follow will help you to put your new knowledge into action, with advice on how to get started. You will learn the actionable steps that you need to take to become the very healthiest version of yourself. I have also included my own personal recommendations for herbal medicine that changed my life and transformed my health. Holistic healing will only work if you do, so ensure that you're taking action on these valuable pieces of advice.

Chapter 9:

Your Current Health Status

Is Your Starting Point

If you're itching to get started on your holistic healing journey, I would advise you to press pause before immediately jumping into treatment. It's great to learn more about your current health status before you start to make decisions on your plans for your health or begin the treatment methods outlined in this book. Learning about where you are right now will clarify how you're able to get to where you want to be. You can't start until you know where you stand right now.

To begin uncovering where you are right now in terms of your health, a great first step is to find a holistic doctor who is a great fit for you. As opposed to going for the first doctor that you find, some research is required to narrow down your choice from the endless options that are out there. While word-of-mouth is great for initial introductions, you should always carry out your own research when selecting a doctor, as what works for someone else may not be appropriate for you.

Step one is to seek out five to ten holistic practitioners that specialize in your condition or the area of your health that you would like to address. With the incredible age of the internet, you are now lucky enough to be able to access international doctors and advice from all over the world. Expand your search and go international, don't just limit yourself to one or two countries. Begin to search for alternative health practitioners or consultants, ensuring that they are licensed. All practitioners will have different backgrounds, so be sure to dig deep and do your research on their website page, getting as many different people's perspectives as possible.

Once you've built a list of five to ten strong contenders that you feel are a good fit, it's great to prepare some questions to ask them. Either set up a consultation call or if you're time-poor, email them over some questions to learn more about them and to see if they have the capabilities to help you in your specific situation. The questions below are designed to assess their credibility, ascertain their relevance to your health problems, and provide a prognosis as to whether they will be able to help you.

What Licenses and/or Certifications Do You Have?

This question should be asked straight off the bat to ensure that the practitioner that you're speaking to is qualified and licensed. You don't want to be taking medical advice from someone who is not a professional. This will help to safeguard your health and give you the reassurance that your health is in the hands of a certified holistic practitioner. Be sure to research the best licenses and certifications that are recognized as being relevant to your condition.

How Long Have You Held Your License?

Selecting a holistic practitioner who has had their license for a long time will give you peace of mind and reassurance. While it's not essential to choose a doctor with decades of experience, it always helps if they have at least a good few years of work under their belt.

What Area(s) Do You Specialize In?

There is little point in seeing a doctor who specializes in cardiovascular holistic healing when you're suffering from gut problems. Holistic doctors often have a specialism, so it's best to make sure that they are fully aligned with your condition. Some may have a more generalized approach, which is great if you're just looking to improve or maintain your overall well-being.

How Will You Diagnose My Health Issues?

It's always best to check what methodologies your holistic doctor uses and to research them to ensure you're comfortable with them. This will also give you an insight into whether they really know their stuff.

What Are the Benefits of Your Suggested Treatment?

When your prospective doctor suggests a treatment, ask what the specific benefits are. It's great to know what you can expect and for them to be able to manage your expectations with regards to the treatment.

What Are the Risks of Your Suggested Treatment?

As with any medicine, it's essential to know the risks. Any good doctor will honestly lay out any risks or side effects that you're likely to experience.

Will This Treatment Interact With Any Medication That I'm Taking?

Make sure that you include any medication that you're currently taking so that the doctor can advise whether it's safe to commence treatment. They will be able to check that your current medication will not cause any problems or adverse reactions and that the treatment will still be effective.

How Long Will the Treatment Take?

It's great to be prepared before considering starting your treatment, so remember to ask the holistic practitioner how long the treatment is likely to take. This will help you to plan and budget for your therapy.

What Is the Success Rate for This Treatment, and Do You Have Any Case Studies?

Asking this question will help you to see if the doctor has tried and tested success with it. Case studies and reviews are also helpful to get some in-depth understanding and context around the situation.

Any reputable professional holistic practitioner should have absolutely no problem answering the questions above. They will appreciate the fact that you have come to the consultation with a desire to take your treatment seriously. It may also be helpful to prepare for some of the common questions that they may ask you. Below are some of the most common questions that holistic practitioners ask prospective clients.

Why Did You Choose to Reach Out to Me?

A holistic doctor will be interested in finding out what your true motivations are for beginning your holistic health journey. As you now know, holistic healing encompasses mental, spiritual, and physical health. You may have some underlying emotional issues that you never considered could be interfering with your physical health. This question will probe you to get to the root of your issue, which will in turn help the doctor recommend an appropriate treatment.

What Are Your Diet and Exercise Currently Like?

The correct nutrition is extremely important to ensure that your holistic treatment works correctly. A good holistic doctor will check that your diet and exercise regime are in top condition and make some suggestions to help you to improve. It may also highlight any areas that you need to work on to improve an imbalance.

What Have You Already Tried?

This question is helpful for several reasons, so do expect to be asked it. The doctor could be about to suggest a treatment that you have already tried but did not work. This will save you both time as they eliminate it from their list of suggestions. It may also identify your personal preferences. If you've tried a strict regime but not been able to stick to it, it suggests that an overly structured approach may not be best for you.

What Are Your Health Concerns?

Your health status is important both for context and for ensuring that you get the correct treatment. Make sure that you discuss all of the concerns that you're having, including any issues like fatigue, pain, or immunity problems. Painting the bigger picture of your health will allow you to receive an ultra-targeted solution.

Often, pinpointing exactly where you are right now with your health can seem difficult and overwhelming. You may not know where to start when describing your health. You may even have difficulty articulating the problem in a way that a doctor could understand. There is no shame in this at all, we all experience very personal manifestations of illness, and it can be hard to communicate this in an efficient way. As long as you're willing to put in some work and make an effort to take steps in the right direction, you will be able to take control of your health. It all starts with being truthful to yourself and getting in touch with yourself regularly.

Start to keep a journal of your health, recording all of the sensations that you're feeling in your body. It's helpful to create daily, weekly, monthly, and yearly recaps of your health to really understand the scope of your well-being. Doing so will help you to identify what your root condition is, as well as provide a holistic perspective of your current condition. Good health isn't achieved as easily as popping a magic pill for an instant solution, staying healthy requires time to adapt to your new healthy habits.

When you're beginning your journaling, observe yourself after you eat and drink and begin to write down how you feel. What did you eat, what time, how quickly, and how did you feel after? You can be as granular in your descriptions as including the ingredients of what you eat if you feel that you're able to. Add in one column with the time and date, then a column with how you feel in yourself after eating and drinking. Do you feel tired, energized, happy, sad, bloated, or satisfied?

All of the contextual elements are important as they will help you to spot patterns and uncover anything that could be an issue. It's time to step up and become your own doctor, as you are the one who should care about yourself the most. After all, nobody knows you better than you!

As well as your eating and drinking habits, journal on how you feel each morning when you wake up, and also before you go to bed. Are you feeling groggy in the morning, or full of energy? Do you find it easy to fall asleep, or do you toss and turn? What activities have you done as you woke up, or as you tried to fall asleep? All of these factors will help you to spot any potential links to your health.

Also, be sure to add in any notable events that may have occurred. You may be able to identify a correlation between specific environments, people, or time periods. The journey to great health is full of discipline, but will eventually lead to an energized life full of vitality and peace. Through the reflection of writing in your journal, you will begin to notice how your body reacts to certain foods and drinks. Sometimes it can be ones that we would have never thought would be an issue. This is a practice that you should adopt for at least two to five years, doing so will cement you as an expert in your own health. Take control of your health, it's a decision that you will never regret.

Chapter 10:

What Are Holistic

Treatment Methods?

As well as working on your diet, mindset, and using herbal medicine for treatment, you may also wish to supplement your health journey with holistic treatment methods. These valuable treatments have been passed down from generation to generation, with their ancient wisdom trusted to treat a range of illnesses and promote general well-being. Many of these treatments have now made their way into the mainstream, with social media popularizing treatments that were once only recognized amongst holistic fanatics' circles. Throughout this chapter, we will examine some of the most popular holistic treatment methods. You will learn what they are, how they are done, and what to expect should you wish to book in for one of them.

Traditional Chinese Medicine

We previously touched on the history of Traditional Chinese Medicine (TCM), it is a holistic health care system that uses a variety of complementary therapies such as acupuncture, moxibustion, massage, *tai chi*, and herbal medicine. As opposed to contemporary Western medicine, which puts emphasis on individual body parts, TCM sees the body as one interconnected whole. According to TCM, your body has interconnected systems that maintain good health through a balance of yin and yang. To achieve optimum health, the body needs to be in a balanced state. Any sickness or disease is linked to an imbalance of your yin and yang energy. TCM seeks to treat whatever the root cause of the imbalance is, which in turn also treats your symptoms too.

To create balance and restore harmony in your body, a TCM practitioner uses a variety of remedies and methods. From cupping to acupuncture, or moxibustion, a TCM healer will evaluate your current health status and provide a recommendation that's tailored to you. A poignant note to make is that one of the cruxes of TCM is the understanding that your body has a life force energy, or *qi,* that is constantly flowing through networks called *meridians.* A TCM practitioner will use several diagnostic methods such as hearing, vibration, voice, touch, and pulse to discover where in your meridians you are experiencing imbalance. From there, they will be able to recommend the appropriate treatment to set you on a path of healing.

Acupuncture and Acupressure

You may be slightly frightened at the thought of having needles inserted into your skin. However, let me reassure you that acupuncture is one of the oldest and most well-respected TCM techniques there is. Acupuncture and acupressure use very thin needles to pierce strategic points on your body. Though it was once used mainly to treat pain, it's now used for stress relief and improvement of general well-being too. The idea behind acupuncture is to balance the *qi* in your body, allowing it to flow freely through the meridians in your body. As the needles are inserted into your meridians, your *qi* will be directed there, allowing your life force energy to balance.

In contrast to many other areas of TCM, this is a practice that many Western doctors actually commend. Modern medicine has recognized the benefits of acupuncture, especially in relation to pain relief. Their view is that the stimulation of nerves and muscles switches on your body's natural painkillers.

Acupuncture is excellent for a range of illnesses and diseases, such as tooth pain, headaches, back pain, osteoporosis, neck pain, and respiratory diseases. Any illnesses that cause you to have chronic pain can also be soothed with regular acupuncture sessions. It is important, however, to note the risks of this procedure. Always ensure that you're visiting a licensed practitioner who is reputable and hygienic. The practitioner should always use sterile or single-use needles and practice good hygiene. If you have any kind of bleeding disorder, a pacemaker, or you are pregnant, you are not a good candidate for acupuncture.

In your first acupuncture session, you can first and foremost expect to have a consultation with the practitioner about your symptoms. They will most likely ask you questions or examine parts of you to uncover which part of your body is painful, such as the rhythm of your pulse, the shape and color of your tongue, and the color of your face. On average, sessions tend to last between 30 and 60 minutes, with a total of six to eight sessions in one treatment plan. The practitioner will ask you to lay on a padded table while they begin to insert needles. The needle may be inserted in a totally different area to where you are experiencing pain or symptoms, but don't worry, this is normal. As the needles are inserted, you shouldn't feel any pain or discomfort, however, you may feel a slight mild ache as the needle reaches the appropriate depth. Once the needles are inserted, the practitioner may manipulate them to stimulate them. This may include twirling or very gently moving the needles. They will remain in place for around ten minutes before being painlessly removed.

After your session, note how you feel. Some people report a boost of energy, whereas others note feeling very calm and relaxed. Record whether your symptoms are getting better after the treatment to ascertain whether acupuncture is the right method for you. An indication that it's working could include less pain, relief of symptoms, or improved overall well-being.

Moxibustion

Moxibustion uses dried plant materials called moxa for heat therapy, burning them on or near the surface of the skin. The idea behind this is to warm your skin, rejuvenating the flow of qi throughout your body. This also helps to remove any toxins or pathogens from your system. Moxa is made up of dried leafy material, often from the Chinese mugwort plant. This herb is excellent to have both in your kitchen cupboard for culinary uses, and in TCM.

There is a range of ailments that moxibustion is excellent at treating. It has been used to treat arthritis, pain from injury, digestive issues, and gynecological problems. It's also excellent as a preventative measure, protecting you against cold and flu illnesses.

As opposed to traditional Chinese practice, holistic practitioners in the U.S tend to hold a stick of burning moxa close to the skin instead of touching it. This is a safer and easier way that often garners the same results. This method uses moxa that's been compressed into a stick or a pole. You may find that this looks similar to a large cigar. The moxa is lit and will then begin to smolder, creating intense heat. The practitioner will then hold the hot moxa stick over a particular area (often ones that correspond to acupuncture points). When the skin of the affected area becomes red and warm, the stick is removed. You may feel a sudden surge of warmth that runs down one of your meridian pathways. This is normal and an indication that the treatment is working correctly. All this signals is that the *qi* has been freed and is now able to flow freely, removing any imbalance.

Tui Na

Tui Na (or Chinese massage therapy) is a form of massage that seeks to balance *qi* by freeing blockages in the body. By removing these blockages, harmony is created in the yin and yang of the body. As blockages often cause illness, disease, and emotional issues, removing them is crucial to overall good health. Just like acupuncture, *Tui Na* focuses on your body's meridians and the flow of *qi*. The main goal is to remove any blocks in your body that may be causing the *qi* to become stagnant.

In a *Tui Na* session, you can expect the massage therapist to use a variety of oscillating and pressure styles that alternate in speed and strength. Depending on your preference and treatment needs, this could be a gentle treatment or a deep-tissue massage. The therapist will massage your muscles using some manipulation techniques that are designed to realign your body and restore optimum function. In *Tui Na*, there are eight techniques used to massage and help the *qi* flow throughout your body:

- Pushing
- Pressing
- Palpating
- Kneading
- Holding
- Lifting

- Rejoining
- Opposing

This wonderful massage technique can be used to treat everything from osteoporosis, arthritis, musculoskeletal disorders, to neck pain, back pain, and digestive conditions. One of its incredible benefits includes the ability to boost blood circulation, as the body's energy flow is stimulated through powerful massage movements. It also has the ability to treat depression. As the focus is on whole-body healing, it has been shown to be effective and provide a therapeutic effect on depression. Astonishingly, it has also been known to improve the quality of life for patients who are suffering from cancer. It's helpful for managing symptoms related to the disease in an alternative way to traditional treatment.

Qigong

If you're looking for an exercise based treatment to incorporate into your healing regime, *qigong* is a marvelous treatment that integrates your mind, body, and spirit. Using breathing techniques, posture, massage, and focused intent, it helps to holistically heal your body. Also known as *Tai Chi*, this holistic healing practice will help to support your long-term health goals.

Just like acupuncture, *qigong* allows *qi* to flow freely throughout the body by opening up the meridian channels. Through regular *qigong* practice, you will notice an enhanced ability to feel life force energy and to connect deeply with it. The movements that *qigong* utilize are slow and gentle, with the aim to warm up your muscles, ligaments and tendons in a safe way. Due to the slower nature of this practice, it's a good low-risk option that you can continue to use as you grow older. Regular *qigong* is known to promote the circulation of your body fluids such as synovial, blood, and lymph. It has also been linked to lowering blood pressure, providing relief from the symptoms of chronic illness, and even assisting with mental disorders and spiritual crises.

A quick internet search should pull up some local *qigong* instructors for you to connect with in your area. If you aren't able to find any local teachers, there are a number of alternatives that you can opt for to try this superb treatment. Head out to a regional or national conference or event to partake in a taster session, you may be able to identify a teacher who is willing to travel to you. Many instructors also carry out online sessions via Skype or Zoom. You could even self-teach, there are excellent videos and books with instructional exercises to get started with. The key is to make sure that you're being consistent with your practice, integrating it into your daily routine to get optimum results.

Chiropractic Treatments

Another of the more mainstream TCM treatments is chiropractic procedures. In chiropractic treatments, your neuromusculoskeletal system including your muscles, nerves, and bones are cared for. A good chiropractor will be able to manage a number of conditions by aligning your spine to create balanced alignment throughout your body. Chiropractic treatments are centered on your body's ability to heal itself, a philosophy that fits nicely into holistic health ideas. In addition to spinal alignment, your chiropractor will also focus on additional treatments such as good nutrition and physical exercise. When you improve your neuromusculoskeletal system, you'll find that other systems in your body are simultaneously improved too.

Ideal for anyone who wants to manage a chronic illness, pain, or simply improve overall well-being, chiropractors can offer improved health without the need to take medication. The amazing benefits that this treatment can offer include the prevention of disease, strengthened immunity, boosted energy, and great holistic well-being. As an average, results are seen in around six to ten visits. Results are achieved through spinal manipulation. A chiropractor will use instruments or their hands to align the joints of the spine. With over 150 different spinal manipulation techniques, your chiropractor will test out a variety of styles to find the one that makes the most positive change for your personal condition. You might hear some popping or cracking sounds as they work, don't worry–this is normal and nothing to panic about.

To supplement the spinal alignment techniques, they may also apply hot and cold treatments, or suggest diet and exercise regimes. Modern chiropractors have even been known to include massage, shoe inserts, and ultrasound therapy to improve their patient's results. You will often receive some tailored advice relevant to your life to take away too, such as posture tips and ways to sit properly at your work desk. Although the most common ailments to visit a chiropractor for include neck and back pain and headaches, chiropractic treatment can also assist arthritis, joint pain, and muscle spasms. Before you book in for your first session, make sure that you've done your homework to ensure that your chosen practitioner is licensed.

Cupping

Although it may look frightening, cupping is a trusted holistic treatment that has been used as a complementary therapy from as long ago as 1550 B.C. Cupping involves placing cups onto your skin to create a suction effect. TCM hails cupping as a way to facilitate healing through improved blood flow. Through cupping, *qi* is stimulated and energy is able to flow freely, filling your body with valuable life force energy. It is excellent for creating balance in the body, removing tension, stimulating cell repair and improving blood flow. Cupping is also used to treat swelling and pain in particular areas as it draws any toxins or impurities to the surface of your skin, allowing them to be easily dispelled. Some people love this treatment so much that they simply use it as a relaxing aid, much in the same way that you would have a massage.

There are a variety of different cupping methods that use different sizes of cups. Smaller cups are ideal for treatment of a small area, whereas larger cups are perfect for a holistic effect, loosening stagnation, and encouraging release of blockages. There are four main techniques that a cupping practitioner may use on you in a treatment session. The first is flash cupping, this is where the cups are squeezed to create a strong suction, before they are placed onto the skin for around 15 minutes before being picked up and then reapplied. This method is great for relief from seasonal flu, sinus issues, and congestion. Another technique is static cupping, where cups are placed and left without movement or manipulation. Water is added to the skin prior to the cup being applied which creates a vacuum-style suction. For any deep tissue problems, shake cupping is used, which uses a shaking or rotation method to manipulate static cups. This works well for softening scars, or for unblocking specific points in your meridian channels. Finally, dynamic cupping uses a sliding motion to slide cups across the surface of your skin. Oil is applied to allow the suction cup to glide, then it is moved in either a circular or diagonal motion across the skin.

You can expect a typical cupping session to last anywhere from 15-60 minutes depending on the treatment technique and the severity of your symptoms. A good practitioner will be able to advise you on how many treatments that you will need to see results for your particular condition. On average, you should begin to see results within five sessions, with the full effect kicking in around ten sessions.

Indian Holistic Treatments

As we explored previously, ancient India provided ideas that underpin many of the concepts and treatments that we see today in modern holistic healing practices. From Ayurveda to yoga, Indian holistic treatments are vastly popular today for both healing and spiritual reasons. Integrating some of the ancient wisdom that India has to offer will help you to create a balanced and well-rounded treatment plan for excellent health.

Ayurveda and Panchakarma

We dived into the history of Ayurveda in Chapter 1, so you are now familiar with its principles and applications. To recap, ayurveda highlights both healing and preventative therapies, marrying science and spirituality to create a holistic system. It takes into account diet, exercise, and living habits to restore balance in the body, preventing disease and restoring health. According to Ayurvedic principles, you are one of three doshas, Vata, Kapha, or Pitta, depending on your own mix of the five basic elements. When your doshic balance is disrupted, it creates imbalance in your body, which in turn creates disease.

For optimum health according to ayurveda, your digestive system, bodily humors, waste products, body tissues, mind, and consciousness must be simultaneously working together in harmony. If the balance between any one of these systems is disrupted, disease will begin to form. In ayurveda, disease is also thought to be a crisis of *ama* toxicity, so to prevent disease, it's important to remove toxins from your body. You can do so by focusing on good nutrition, exercise, and through cleansing techniques like *panchakarma.*

Panchakarma is the process of purification, helping you to destress and remove toxins, or *ama,* from your body. Depending on your own dosha or disorder, an ayurvedic practitioner will be able to recommend one of the five following panchakarma methods.

The first panchakarma method used is emesis therapy. This is superb for any kind of respiratory illness, or viruses such as colds and flu. These types of illnesses are characterized by an excess of mucus signal over-indexing in kapha. The Ayurvedic treatment ritual for this is therapeutic vomiting, or *vamana.* This eliminates the excess mucus and can also help to rid the body of repressed emotions that lurk in the kapha areas of the stomach and lungs. An instant sense of relief can be felt and you should be able to breathe freely afterwards with significantly reduced congestion. This method should always be practiced under the advice or supervision of an ayurvedic professional.

The next technique of panchakarma is purgation therapy, this uses a therapeutic laxative to help purge the system of toxins. Excess bile in your system can wreak havoc, causing issues as it's secreted into the gallbladder with problems like inflammation, rashes, acne, fever, and nausea appearing. This is thought to be due to an excess of pitta in the body. Purgatives can help to resolve or completely fix these issues, as well as eating foods designed to balance the excess pitta.

When there is a vata imbalance and the body begins to have too much vata, enema therapy is recommended to restore balance. Vata is often thought to be the main culprit in the manifestation of illness and disease in ayurvedic practice. Medicine administered rectally is able to reach deeper into tissues and bones. This corrects a variety of issues such as bone problems, fluid retention, and the majority of diseases. Again, this should always be undertaken with the help of a professional.

Ayurveda recognizes the nose as the doorway to the brain, and therefore, to your consciousness. In nasya therapy, medication is administered nasally, eliminating any issues with your nose, throat, sinus, or head. This treatment is able to improve breathing, congestion, and migraines. As the medication is inserted into the nose, a light massage is used to ensure that the treatment is as deep and effective as possible. Any emotions that have been trapped in the respiratory tract are released, which also helps physical parts of your body such as your eyes. Be sure to keep your fingernails short and to apply the medication gently to prevent injury of your delicate nasal passage.

Finally, rakta moksha is sometimes used as a method of purifying and cleansing the blood. This is a traditional ayurvedic treatment that should only be carried out by a professional. Also known as 'bloodletting,' this style of treatment includes extracting a very small amount of blood from a vein to relieve tension. This stimulates the spleen, forcing it to produce anti-toxic and immune stimulating substances. This then neutralizes any toxins in the blood, promoting purification and good health. This type of treatment is ideal for repetitive conditions such as eczema, acne, herpes, and hives, as well as liver and spleen problems. Of course, please do not attempt to try this treatment yourself, this should only be carried out by a licensed practitioner.

Yoga

Yoga is often practiced for physical benefits in the Western world, however, yoga has astonishing health benefits when used in conjunction with other holistic treatments. Yoga is an excellent way to not only promote mental and spiritual wellness, but to offer a retreat from chronic illnesses and diseases. Incorporating yoga into your routine will create holistic health benefits for your mind, body, and energy. There is often a common misconception that yoga is difficult or painful. Yoga does not have to include complicated positions, simply trying out simple poses and setting some daily time aside for your practice will ensure that you're still reaping all of the benefits.

From improving your flexibility (which prevents pain), upgrading your joint health, and promoting better breathing, yoga will have demonstrable results on your physical health. As you spend more time sitting at desks and in front of your devices, yoga also helps to prevent back pain and decompress your spine. The mental calmness and de-stressing capabilities of yoga have also been tied to assisting mental disorders like anxiety and depression.

Indian Homeopathy

Homeopathic medicine is one of the predominant holistic healing methods used in India (alongside Ayurveda). In synchronicity with holistic healing principles, it focuses on the balancing of mind, body and spirit for optimum health. Rather than putting the spotlight on the treatment and management of symptoms, it provides safe medication for long-term use to prevent sickness and create lasting optimum health.

Homeopathy itself is a form of holistic medicine that uses very diluted substances to activate your body's healing powers. The substances include a mix of plants, minerals, and other natural substances designed to stimulate your body's natural healing process. In contrast to contemporary medicine, the aim is to heal your body permanently, faster, and for a less-expensive cost. Fans of homeopathy include Mahatma Gandhi and Dr. Deepak Chopra. Interestingly, the more that a homeopathic treatment is diluted, the stronger its healing properties become.

Treatment will begin by identifying what symptoms or problems you're currently facing, with the appropriate homeopathic remedy provided to restore balance in your body. Unlike chemical treatments, homeopathic remedies work well for issues that are caused by a lack of balance, such as emotional and psychological disorders. To find a homeopathic doctor or hospital, conduct an internet search and be sure to read online reviews and case studies on doctors that interest you.

Further Holistic Treatment Methods

The treatment methods below comprise a combination of both modern and traditional therapies. They are excellent additions to your holistic healing routine and may be used alone, or in conjunction with any of the treatment methods outlined in this chapter.

Reflexology

Reflexology with a certified massage therapist is an excellent way to receive a holistic treatment that also feels like a relaxing treat at the same time! Taking time to unwind and experience a massage will do your physical and mental health a world of good. Reflexology uses an application of pressure by the masseuse to specific areas on your feet or hands. This treatment is designed to relieve stress and relax you, with the pressure applied to particular pressure points on your foot as they correspond with different areas of your body.

As the masseuse applies pressure to certain spots, relaxation and healing is flooded to the corresponding organ or area of your body. Using detailed foot charts, reflexologists will be guided to the specific area that you need. This treatment technique is ideal for the reduction of pain, stress, insomnia and anxiety.

Reiki

Reiki is an ancient Japanese holistic treatment method that has long been used to promote healing, stress relief, and relaxation. The idea behind Reiki is for a practitioner to use their hands to move and balance the life force energy in your body. As you know, when life force energy is balanced, you're more likely to be healthy and to prevent or heal disease. During a reiki session, a practitioner will use their hands to deliver life force energy to your body, in turn promoting healing.

Reiki is wonderful for energetically balancing your body, and has been known to stimulate your immune system, relieve pain, promote self-healing, and support any contemporary medication that you might be taking. During a session, you may also feel a strong sense of calmness, security, and relaxation. Many describe the sensation of reiki as a glowing, warm energy or radiance that flows to and through you from the practitioner's hands.

Reports indicate that as well as helping to balance your mind, body, and spirit, reiki assists with a range of conditions such as cancer, infertility, pain, digestive issues and mental health conditions. This safe and effective method is great to use alongside any traditional or other holistic treatments that you may be undertaking.

Aromatherapy

As well as smelling wonderful, aromatherapy treatment techniques have powerful results that can help with a range of mild to serious conditions. Aromatherapists are trained in the science of aromas, using plant aromas to heal and treat sickness and disease. With regular aromatherapy treatments, you're able to unlock a more balanced state of health. From the treatment of conditions, to improved relaxation and sleep, aromatherapy is an excellent therapeutic method.

You may wish to visit an aromatherapist for mild issues such as a cold or flu, or for general skin conditions. A certified aromatherapist can also help with more serious ailments, like arthritis, high blood pressure, parasites, or fibromyalgia. As with many other holistic treatments, an aromatherapist practitioner will talk with you to uncover your symptoms, medical history, and any medications that you're currently taking. From there, they will be able to create your very own signature blend, formulated to treat your specific concerns. Most aromatherapists will even allow you to test and smell the aroma, making sure it's to your personal liking.

From there, they will provide you with a treatment plan that instructs you on when and how to take your blend. There are several ways to administer an aromatherapy blend, from vaporizers, to steamers and diffusers. In certain cases, the aromatherapist will instruct you to massage the oil into your skin, or even ingest it, however, this should always be done at the discretion of a professional. After a treatment plan is created, the aromatherapist will keep in touch with you to ensure that the blend is meeting all of your health goals, or if the formula needs to be tweaked.

Holistic Nutritionist

As nutrition is such a vital part of holistic health, it can be helpful to seek the help of a holistic nutritionist, especially if you are new to all things holistic. Although it seems overwhelming at first when looking to completely overhaul your diet, with some help to point you in the right direction, your transition to a natural diet shouldn't be too difficult.

A holistic nutritionist is a specialist who teaches you how to use natural and organic food to holistically improve your whole body. The focus is on improving your mental, physical, and emotional state through the consumption of nutritional foods. When you consult a holistic nutritionist, they will offer you everything from a nutritious meal plan, to tips and advice on living a healthy lifestyle in general.

You can expect a holistic nutritionist to begin with a deep dive into your current eating habits, food choices, and lifestyle. They will also seek to identify any potential stressors or triggers. From there, they will be able to develop a personalized meal plan and food shopping list, enabling you to make informed and healthy choices. The foods that they suggest should be non-GMO, organic, natural, and free from additives and preservatives. Although they will be able to help make suggestions, it is ultimately down to you to ensure that you stick to the plan and follow through. Try to keep a food journal and motivate yourself throughout this process, as it will only work if you do.

Kinesiology

A final therapeutic practice to consider is kinesiology. This therapy takes into consideration the skeletal and muscular systems, looking at how they relate both to each other and to diseases. Not to be confused with physiotherapy, kinesiology focuses on medical conditions and strengthening the body, as opposed to physiotherapy which focuses on injury and rehabilitation.

In essence, kinesiology is the study of body movements. A kinesiologist will focus on which one of your body parts is functioning incorrectly. They will attempt to strengthen your musculoskeletal system holistically to treat it and prevent any future issues. The benefits of kinesiology include the reduction of healing time for chronic illnesses, and the reduction of any pain associated with them. A kinesiologist will be able to quickly identify any of your muscles and bones that aren't functioning properly and work to improve them. As your skeletal and muscular systems are so delicate, please ensure that you only visit a licensed kinesiologist.

Chapter 11:

Author Experience and

Tips

Over the 25 years that I have been on my own holistic healing journey, I have tried just about every single holistic treatment that there is. Some have not worked, some did not have the desired effect, but some have been absolutely instrumental in my health. I am proud and excited to share my favorite treatments with you. These are the treatments that from my experience should be a staple in any holistic enthusiast's cupboards, the ones that I always recommend to friends, and the ones that I still use to this day.

Wild Chaga Tea

I first discovered the magic of *Chaga* when I found myself suffering from a sore throat. All of the over-the-counter remedies that I tried had never worked, and as I was converting to holistic treatments, I began to research alternatives. When I discovered *Chaga*, I learned that not only is it excellent at treating sore throats, but it can also aid colds and help to reduce coughing. I wasn't sure what to expect when I took it, but as soon as I tried it using a tincture method, I experienced immediate effects. I had increased energy, as if I had just drunk a large coffee, but without the crash that I used to suffer from afterward. My sore throat disappeared and I felt soothed and healed straight away, unlike anything that I had ever experienced before.

As you embark on your holistic healing journey, you may experience a sneaky craving from time to time for a wine or beer. I always make sure that I keep this tea around the house, or on my person when traveling to use as an alternative to alcohol. This is one of the main factors that I attribute to my incredible health. Of course, be sure to consult your doctor before taking *Chaga*, as everyone's health condition is unique to them, and I cannot generalize a treatment.

Chaga is a mushroom, it is a non-toxic fungus that can be found on birch and a range of other trees. This magical mushroom has several benefits and medicinal qualities, which makes it popular for use in herbal healing. Although it doesn't look very appealing (it has a burnt charcoal-like appearance), it contains qualities that heal and strengthen the body naturally. *Chaga* is one of the oldest, safest, yet most powerful herbal treatments that there is. One of the properties that makes *Chaga* so effective is its makeup being packed full of antioxidants. *Chaga* contains 36,557 ORAC (oxygen radical absorbance capacity) per 1g. This is miles more than foods that are often hailed as antioxidant powerhouses such as goji berries (400 ORAC PER 1g), acai berries (800 ORAC per 1g), and blueberries (24.5 ORAC per 1g). It also contains over 215 phytonutrients as it is naturally occurring and not synthetic. Consume your *Chaga* in tea, or opt for a tincture, which is my preferred method of consumption.

Wild Ban Lan Gen Tea

My secret weapon for the winter season is *Ban Lan Gen* tea (also known as Isatis Tinctoria). This lesser-known tea has provided me with remarkable results. I always keep plenty in stock for the fall and winter seasons. Unlike *Chaga* tea, it does not provide an energy boost, instead, it has more of a soothing and relaxing effect. This tea is the one that I reach for to relieve inflammation from my sore throat, eliminate cold and flu, and cease coughing straight away. I was pleasantly surprised to get immediate results from drinking this tea in a steaming hot mug. One side-effect that annoyed me at first was that it made me need the toilet quite a lot. Once I realized why this was though, I was more than happy to make a couple of extra trips to the restroom. *Ban Lan Gen* tea is so good at expelling toxins from your body, that it will cause you to urinate them out at a frequent rate. Better out than in, right? You'll notice the color of your urine turns from dark to light throughout the day as the tea filters all of the toxins out of your body.

One benefit of this tea is that it costs considerably less than *Chaga* tea, so it's ideal if you're on a tight budget. This is due to the abundance of it in nature. If you're ready to kiss goodbye to your seasonal colds and illnesses, this tea is for you. As always, please make sure that you consult a licensed holistic doctor before consuming *Ban Lan Gen* tea, as your health condition is unique and requires tailored advice.

Ban Lan Gen is a root that's been used for centuries, especially in TCM (traditional Chinese medicine). This root is also known as woad, dyer's woad, indigowoad root, and *Da Qing Ye*, so keep an eye out for these variations of the name when shopping for this tea. The ingredient is traditionally grown in Asian countries such as Japan and China, as well as various tropical countries worldwide. The roots are turned into powder, capsules, and tea, ready to be drunk by consumers to heal their bodies. It's safe to consume tea three to four times in one day, however, it's best to limit consumption to a maximum of seven days to avoid side effects. As well as the sore throat, cold, and cough healing mentioned earlier, *Ban Lan Gen* tea is excellent for aiding a number of other conditions.

This tea is famed for being able to help with respiratory conditions such as congested lungs, pneumonia, and bronchitis. It is also extremely powerful as an antiviral and antibacterial aid. However, use it with caution, as it is so potent that it can kill good bacteria too. My advice would be to take it alongside some probiotics to offset this. The antiviral properties are great at assisting with illnesses like mumps, measles, chickenpox, herpes, psoriasis, and tonsillitis too. As it has strong anti-inflammatory properties, it can also soothe pain related to arthritis, gout, and inflammation of the limbs and spine.

Heat your *Ban Lan Gen* tea in your favorite mug, adding a little natural sweetener such as honey if you require it. Consume this several times a day for the best effects, but remember to only use it on a seven-day cycle under guidance from your holistic doctor.

Organic Yerba Mate

Yerba mate has been my go-to tea for daily consumption throughout my holistic healing journey. Rather than standard green tea, this antioxidant powerhouse will provide you with far better results. My experience with this tea has been amazing, as its immune-boosting, anti-inflammatory, and antioxidant properties work like no other. This tea provides a much-needed energy boost and gives me razor-sharp mental focus. Another great bonus is that drinking this tea regularly will help to reduce any excess tummy fat—this is exactly what happened to me. I love to drink this tea all day long, it's delicious and convenient. I would recommend substituting your usual coffee for this tea each morning, as traditional coffee has a lot of toxins that your body could do without. Please make sure that you check in with your holistic doctor to ensure it's safe to consume alongside your treatment regime.

Yerba tea is a herbal tea that utilizes the leaves and twigs of a plant called Ilex Paraguariensis. Traditionally, the leaves are dried over a fire and steeped in water to make the delicious tea. It is usually drunk from a container that's called a 'gourd' and sipped with a metal straw with a filter to prevent you from drinking any fragments of leaf. This wonderful tea is packed full of transformative benefits.

It is an antioxidant powerhouse, containing several plant nutrients such as saponins (anti-inflammatory), xanthines (natural stimulants), caffeoyl (anti-oxidants), and polyphenols (disease preventers). As I mentioned before, yerba mate contains more antioxidant power than green tea, which is often hailed as the healthiest tea. This tea is packed full of seven out of the nine essential amino acids and also boasts nearly all of the vitamins and minerals that your body needs. It is also known for being able to give you an energy boost. You will feel less tired, as well as have the ability to focus more and experience true mental clarity. You can expect to have the alertness of coffee without the crash or jitters.

Yerba mate has antibacterial properties that prevent illness from parasites, fungi, and many kinds of bacteria. It can even be a remedy for sickness like E.coli and food poisoning, reducing stomach cramps, sickness, and diarrhea. Drinking regular yerba mate also gives your immune system a welcome boost, due to its high vitamin C, E, zinc, and selenium content. The antioxidant properties are also linked to protection against heart disease and support for your cardiovascular system.

To prepare your yerba mate tea, fill a calabash or french press with dried or toasted leaves and add hot water. For taste, feel free to add in some stevia, lemon, or honey. Even though most people drink this tea hot, you can serve it as a cold beverage over ice if you prefer.

Organic Peppermint Tea

You've probably heard about peppermint tea before, but don't overlook this impressive tea just because it's common. Rather than stimulating your body life coffee, and peppermint tea are known to relax the nervous system. I found that this tea really helped my digestive system and reduced symptoms like bloating and stomach pain. As most of us don't eat properly, this gives the digestive system a helping hand. My experience using peppermint tea has always been fantastic. I don't get any headaches or migraines anymore as long as I'm regularly drinking this tea. Before you stock up your cupboards, make sure that you run it past your holistic doctor, just in case.

There are so many great benefits to peppermint tea. It is an all-around soother, helping you to have a restful night's sleep, aiding your digestion, and relieving stress. It even has the power to eliminate bad breath, create mental alertness, and boost your immune system.

In terms of digestion, we could all use a helping hand from time to time. Our bodies are always working overtime to digest our food, so anything that we can do to assist it will help to improve your overall health. Peppermint tea relaxes the digestive tract and allows bile to properly flow, keeping your digestion functioning well at all times. It also creates a passage for gas to travel through the body, releasing any trapped wind to aid bloating, flatulence, and stomach pain. In the process of this, it will also maintain a steady rhythm to your bowel movements which can stop hemorrhoids from forming. If you suffer from IBS, you should look to consume peppermint tea several times a day. Peppermint tea soothes the gastrointestinal tract, which is where many of the IBS symptoms originate. It even has the power to activate a channel in the colon which can alleviate pain and soothe inflammation.

Some more of the wonderful uses for peppermint tea include its ability to relieve stress and soothe your mental state. The menthol that's found in the tea is a sedative and also has muscle relaxing properties. As soon as you have a sip, its body and mind relaxation effects will kick in, allowing you to destress fully. It's also able to reduce your blood pressure, and for this reason, peppermint essential oils are often used in complementary therapies such as massage. If you choose to have a cup of peppermint tea before bedtime you'll notice that it will help to improve your sleep. If you suffer from insomnia, it's a great idea to drink a cup before you go to sleep. The menthol in the peppermint leaves will help your muscles to relax and allow you to drift off into a deep sleep.

You're able to consume peppermint tea at any time of the day. Consumed in the morning, it will allow you to harness its mental focus improving qualities. If you choose to drink it during the day, it will help with digestion, or have a cup at night-time for a great night's sleep. I would recommend drinking around two to three cups a day. Always go for fresh peppermint leaves as opposed to store-bought variants so that you know that no sneaky synthetic chemicals are lurking in your drink. Add one tablespoon of chopped peppermint leaves to boiling water, allowing it to steep for five minutes before draining.

I'm so excited for you to begin using these treatments and reaping the wonderful benefits of my favorite recommendations. These four treatments are all in liquid form, so they should be easy and accessible for you to get started with. As with all things, the potency of each and how much you should consume varies for each individual person. As I always say, it's best to consult a licensed holistic practitioner to ensure that you're advised on the correct dosage for your personal health needs.

Chapter 12:

So, What's Next? Recap and Author Thoughts

You have learned so much about holistic health and how to step up and take control of your own health. You should be feeling inspired, motivated, and ready to become the very healthiest version of yourself. Although it may seem overwhelming at first, you now have all the knowledge that you need at your fingertips, always accessible in this book whenever you may need it. If you're wondering if this information will give you the results that you want, the answer is yes, absolutely–as long as you first learn about your own health, and realize that work is required to get the result that you so badly want.

This information has been around for thousands of years, with millions of proven success stories. First, you need to acknowledge that you need to embark on a journey to truly know yourself. Follow the exercises in this book such as journaling to get in touch with your own health and learn about your body. Then start to apply the history and holistic principles to your own health, realizing that this is the beginning of changing yourself. Knowing your current health status is the key to unlocking optimum health, you can't get to where you want to be without knowing where you currently are. Your best source of information is yourself, so ensure that you're taking time to get in touch with your body and record it in your personal journal.

Use the advice given on pollution to evaluate how clean the air that you're breathing is. Clean air matters as pure oxygen is vital to healing and keeping you healthy. Although this sounds like common sense to most people, the air that we breathe is something that we're likely to give little thought to. Have you ever purchased an air freshener for your home or car? As lovely as these are, these products are toxic. These smells are not natural or organic, and breathing them in is inviting toxins into your system. Reading labels and using only organic material is key to understanding your body and how it can become affected by external items. A great transition for me was to throw away all of the synthetic air fresheners in my home and go into the forest for one or two weeks at a time. I love to camp, and I found that being in the fresh air without any pollution or chemicals was a wonderful reset for my body. Try it– your body will love you for it! You'll notice immediate results as you remove yourself from all of the toxins in the city air. See this as reverting back to the lifestyle that our healthy, ancient ancestors lived.

You're reading this book as you want to take action. Taking action will allow you to get a new result. Remember that your health is your responsibility, not your doctor's. Although it's great to have a wonderful doctor who can assist and advise you, at the end of the day, you will need the discipline to see through all of the recommendations that they provide. With holistic doctors, there should always be two-way communication. Make sure that you're providing enough context and dialogue so that they can constantly give you the best advice. Ensure that you follow their advice fully and complete any of the treatment plans that they give to you. Your body is changing daily, so no one medicine will fix you instantly. You're committing yourself to be in it for the long run. My journey to having unlimited health has been long and challenging. Of course, there were times that I wanted to give up. There were times when it was hard, but I never gave up. The results that I achieved are more than worth the sacrifices that I made. This book is just the tip of the iceberg when it comes to rebalancing the body.

You don't have to become overwhelmed and try everything all at once. As humans, we take a long time to build habits. My advice would be to start in small steps. Try the smaller tasks and swaps to get yourself on the right track without wanting to throw in the towel too early. Believe in yourself, and affirm that you can do it. Start to change your lifestyle by drinking herbal tea to rebalance any imbalances in your body. Swap out drinks that you're currently consuming and try the teas that I have suggested in the previous chapter. Most people will simply read the information in this book and not take action, but I challenge you to do the opposite. Take immediate action. Start with the recommended teas, as this is a quick and easy first step. You'll begin to enjoy them in no time and before you know it, they'll be integrated into part of your daily routine.

All of the elements have the potential to affect your body. Air affects your body the fastest, hence my recommendations about taking regular breaks in the fresh air. Water also affects your blood, but this can take some time. Earth and solid matter take even longer to get into your blood, but they can cause havoc when it does. In my experience, many people don't think about the things that we consume on a daily basis and how they affect our health. I would like you to consider everything from now on. How are the things that you breathe, drink, and eat affecting you and your health? What changes could you make? What would the results be? Remember to look at the bigger picture of your health. This is exactly what holistic healing is all about. You need to uncover the root cause of your illness, which is done by assessing your current health status. Then you can use your newfound knowledge of organic, natural herbs to heal and treat your conditions and maintain perfect health.

I have loved sharing my knowledge with you in this book. I have every confidence in you and I know that you will be taking empowered steps to take back control of your health from the moment that you finish this book. If you think that you have learned something beneficial, I would absolutely love for you to support my next book by taking one or two minutes of your time to leave a short review on Amazon. I would appreciate all of your feedback and positive thoughts. My passion is to give people the incredible results that I have had for many years without any biased information. I hope that I have achieved this, and I wish you all of the best in your holistic healing journey. Thank you.

Glossary

Acidic Diet: A diet high in acidic foods such as meat and dairy.

Acupuncture: A holistic treatment where very thin needles are inserted into the skin to promote the flow of life force energy.

Ailment: A type of illness or sickness, often a minor one.

Air Pollutant: Any physical, biological, or chemical agent containing toxins that is emitted into the air.

Alkaline Diet: A diet high in alkaline foods such as certain fruit and vegetables.

Allopathic Medicine: A modern system of treatment by healthcare professionals that focuses on the use of treating symptoms with drugs.

Anatomist: Someone who has expert knowledge about anatomy.

Aromatherapy: The use of the aromas of plants for therapeutic healing purposes.

Astringent: A substance that causes skin cells to contract.

Ayurveda: An ancient Indian system of medicine that seeks to balance the body using holistic methods.

Ban Lan Gen: A traditional Chinese medicine that is often consumed in tea as a remedy for virus-related diseases.

Bile: A bitter, alkaline fluid that is secreted by the liver.

Biomolecular: Substances that are created by living organisms.

BMI: Body mass index. A tool used to measure height and weight to indicate health.

Capsaicin: A compound that is found in spicy food that gives the sensation of heat.

Carcinogen: Any substance that has the ability to cause cancer.

Carrier Oil: An oil made from plants that are often used to dilute other more potent oils.

Chaga: A fungus found on birch that has antioxidant properties that are beneficial to health.

Chiropractor: A holistic practitioner that treats misalignment of the joints.

Confucius: A sixth-century Chinese philosopher.

Contemporary Medicine: Modern, Western medical practices.

Cupping: A Chinese medical treatment where heated cups are applied to the skin to create free-flowing life force energy.

Doshas: Three forms of substances that are present in every person's body and mind, and that cause problems when imbalanced.

Emesis Therapy: An Ayurvedic therapeutic vomiting treatment.

Enema Therapy: An Ayurvedic liquid treatment administered rectally.

Energetics: The properties of something in terms of the energy that it has.

Essential Oil: A distilled oil taken from plants or natural materials.

Galen: A Greek anatomist who developed theories on the way that the human body functions.

Genetically Modified: A crop that has been artificially modified to create desired features and characteristics.

Herbal Combinations: A mix of several different herbs used to produce a prescription to treat illness.

Herbal Decoction: An extraction method used to extract nutrients from bark and roots.

Herbal Infusion: A concoction made from steeping herbs in water or oil until the nutrients are absorbed.

Herbal Medicine: Medicine and treatments that use active ingredients from herbs and plants.

Herbal Ointment: Therapeutic balms or salves that are administered topically.

Herbal Poultice: A paste made of herbs with specific healing properties.

Herbal Tincture: Herbal medicine that is administered through a small dropper bottle.

Herbalism: The study of the medicinal purpose of plants.

Hippocrates: A Greek physician who studied and taught medicine.

Holism: The theory that different parts are all interconnected and part of the same whole.

Holistic Health: An approach that takes into consideration the whole person, as opposed to just their individual parts.

Holistic Medicine: A form of medicine that considers the complete person, taking into consideration mental, physical, and spiritual factors.

Homeopathy: A treatment that uses minute doses of a substance to treat illness and disease.

Inflammation: The process of white blood cells protecting the body from illness as an immune response.

Kapha: An Ayurvedic dosha that is based on air and water. Those with Kapha doshas are often big-boned, large, strong, and caring.

Kinesiology: A study into the mechanics of the musculoskeletal system.

Life Force Energy: The energy that exists in all living beings and is responsible for their vitality.

Mainstream Medicine: Conventional Western medicine that focuses on the use of drugs and surgery to treat disease and sickness.

Meridians: The set of interconnected pathways throughout the body that life force energy is able to flow through.

Moxibustion: A Traditional Chinese therapy where a practitioner burns a plant called moxa near the patient's skin to restore their flow of life force energy.

Nasya Therapy: An Ayurvedic treatment that utilizes the application of medicine through the nasal passage.

Noxious Gasses: A poisonous gas that can be harmful or deadly if ingested.

Oxidative Stress: When the balance between antioxidants and free radicals in the body occurs.

Ozone: An unstable toxic gas often formed through ultraviolet light.

Panchakarma: Ayurvedic methods of cleansing and purging the body of toxins.

Particulate Matter: Solid or liquid particles in the air that can be dangerous if ingested.

Pathogen: A virus that can cause disease and sickness.

Pitta: An Ayurvedic dosha that is based on fire and water. Those with Pitta doshas are often athletic, competitive, muscular, and tenacious.

Prakruti: An Ayurvedic term for anything in its natural condition.

Prana: The universal energy flow that streams throughout the body, such as in breath.

Pulmonary Ventilation: The process of air flowing through the lungs to facilitate oxygen absorption and carbon dioxide excretion.

Purgation Therapy: An Ayurvedic treatment used to cleanse the body with the therapeutic use of laxatives.

Qi: A Traditional Chinese term for life force energy.

Qigong: A Traditional Chinese movement also known as Tai Chi.

Rakta Moksha: An Ayurvedic treatment that aims to remove toxins from the body through bloodletting.

Reflexology: A massage system that focuses on specific points on the hands or feet to relieve sickness and disease.

Reiki: A Japanese healing technique used to channel energy into the patient to promote self-healing.

Stevia: A calorie-free, natural sugar substitute.

Toxin: A poison that acts as an antigen in the body.

Traditional Chinese Medicine: An ancient system of health and wellness that has been used for thousands of years in China.

Tui Na: A Traditional Chinese form of massage that is used to treat illness.

Vata: An Ayurvedic dosha that is based on air and space. Those with Vata doshas are often energetic, free, lively, and creative.

Vedas: Ancient Indian scriptures that include Ayurveda.

Vikruti: Translated from Sanskrit as "after creation." A human's biological constitution, referring to their state of health.

Volatile Organic Compounds: Organic chemicals that have a high vapor pressure.

Yerba Mate: A South American herb used in therapeutic tea that's known to improve health through its high antioxidant content.

Yoga: A spiritual discipline that is practiced for health, relaxation, and optimum health.

References

1MD. (2022). *High Stress: Symptoms, Causes, Complications, and Treatment*. 1MD. https://1md.org/health-guide/heart/symptoms/high-stress

Adams, C. (2014, January 2). *Natural vs. Synthetic Vitamins – What's the Big Difference?* Sunwarrior; Sunwarrior. https://sunwarrior.com/blogs/health-hub/natural-vs-synthetic-vitamins

Afshin, A. (2019). Health effects of dietary risks in 195 countries, 1990–2017: a systematic analysis for the Global Burden of Disease Study 2017. *The Lancet*, *393*(10184), 1958–1972.

https://www.sciencedirect.com/science/article/
pii/S0140673619300418

Agócs, R., Sugár, D., & Szabó, A. J. (2020). Is too
much salt harmful? Yes. *Pediatric Nephrology
(Berlin, Germany)*, 35(9), 1777–1785.
https://doi.org/10.1007/s00467-019-04387-4

Argosy Publishing, Inc. (2018). *5 Functions of
Respiratory System.* Visiblebody.com.
https://www.visiblebody.com/learn/respiratory
/5-functions-of-respiratory-system

Ayurvedic India. (2007, September 22). *What Is
Ayurveda? The History Of Ayurveda.*
Ayurvedic   India.
https://www.ayurvedicindia.info/history-of-
ayurveda/

Azaïs-Braesco, V., Sluik, D., Maillot, M., Kok, F., &
Moreno, L. A. (2017). A review of total &

added sugar intakes and dietary sources in Europe. *Nutrition Journal*, *16*(1), 6. https://doi.org/https://doi.org/10.1186/s12937-016-0225-2

B, N. (2019, August 15). *How To Achieve Self Empowerment?* TheMindFool - Perfect Medium for Self-Development & Mental Health. Explorer of Lifestyle Choices & Seeker of the Spiritual Journey. https://themindfool.com/steps-you-can-take-to-achieve-self-empowerment/

Bauer, B. (2018). *Reflexology for stress relief.* Mayo Clinic. https://www.mayoclinic.org/healthy-lifestyle/consumer-health/expert-answers/what-is-reflexology/faq-20058139

Berliner, H. S., & Salmon, J. W. (1980). The Holistic Alternative to Scientific Medicine: History and Analysis. *International Journal of Health Services*, *10*(1), 133–147. https://doi.org/10.2190/xwr6-5qpx-gege-5gwr

Body, V. (2022). *5 Functions of Respiratory System | Respiratory Anatomy*. Www.visiblebody.com. https://www.visiblebody.com/learn/respiratory /5-functions-of-respiratory-system#:~:text=External%20Respiration%20E xchanges%20Gases%20Between

Brennan, D. (2021). *What Is a Chiropractor?* WebMD. https://www.webmd.com/a-to-z-guides/what-is-chiropractor

Brody, J. E. (1983, September 21). EATING SPICY FOOD: WHAT ARE THE EFFECTS? *The New York Times*. https://www.nytimes.com/1983/09/21/garden/

eating-spicy-food-what-are-the-
effects.html?pagewanted=all

Butler, N. (2018, July 24). *Are acidic foods harmful to health?* Www.medicalnewstoday.com. https://www.medicalnewstoday.com/articles/3 22557#evidence

Cacioppo, J. T., & Patrick, W. (2008). *Loneliness human nature and the need for social connection.* New York Norton.

Calabro, S. (2009, August 25). *Alternative Medicine Pros and Cons.* EverydayHealth.com. https://www.everydayhealth.com/alternative-health/the-basics/are-you-conisdering-complementary-and-alternative-medicine.aspx

Caldwell, P. (2022). *Tinctures - What are they and how do you use them? | Herb Lore.*

Herblore.com. https://herblore.com/overviews/tinctures

Canadian Mental Health Association. (2008). *The Relationship between Mental Health, Mental Illness and Chronic Physical Conditions | CMHA Ontario.* Cmha.ca. https://ontario.cmha.ca/documents/the-relationship-between-mental-health-mental-illness-and-chronic-physical-conditions/

Chaga Mountain. (2022). *What is chaga - Chaga Mountain, Inc.* Chagamountain.com. https://chagamountain.com/what-is-chaga/

Cleveland Clinic. (2020, January 24). *Respiratory System: Functions, Facts, Organs & Anatomy.* Cleveland Clinic; Cleveland Clinic. https://my.clevelandclinic.org/health/articles/21205-respiratory-system

Cleveland Clinic. (2021, September 13). *Cardiovascular System: Overview, Anatomy and Function.* Cleveland Clinic. https://my.clevelandclinic.org/health/body/218 33-cardiovascular-system

Cloverleaf Farm. (2011, January 9). *Ointments and Salves - Herbal Encyclopedia.* Www.cloverleaffarmherbs.com. https://www.cloverleaffarmherbs.com/modes-of-use/ointments-and-salves/

Cold-Q. (2016, August 19). *Benefits of Herbal Medicine You Need to Know.* Cold-Q™. https://coldq.com/benefits-of-herbal-medicine-you-need-to-know/

Cole, S. (2021, November 9). *The Benefits Of Herbal Medicine.* The Healthcare Guys.

https://www.healthcareguys.com/2021/11/09/the-benefits-of-herbal-medicine/

D'Elia, L., Galletti, F., & Strazzullo, P. (2014). Dietary salt intake and risk of gastric cancer. *Cancer Treatment and Research, 159*(6), 83–95.

D'Elia, L., Rossi, G., Ippolito, R., Cappuccio, F. P., & Strazzullo, P. (2012). Habitual salt intake and risk of gastric cancer: A meta-analysis of prospective studies. *Clinical Nutrition, 31*(4), 489–498. https://doi.org/10.1016/j.clnu.2012.01.003

Davies, J. (2017, June 18). *10 Negative Coping Mechanisms People Use to Hide from Their Problems*. Learning Mind. https://www.learning-mind.com/coping-mechanisms/

Dr. Chuanxin Wang - OM Clinical / Faculty Supervisor. (2017). *Acupuncture and Massage College*. Acupuncture and Massage College. https://www.amcollege.edu/blog/the-essential-elements-that-define-holistic-health

Dyer, M. H. (2022). *StackPath*. Www.gardeningknowhow.com. https://www.gardeningknowhow.com/edible/herbs/hgen/homemade-poultice-for-healing.htm

Edwards, S. J., Montgomery, I. M., Colquhoun, E. Q., Jordan, J. E., & Clark, M. G. (1992). Spicy meal disturbs sleep: an effect of thermoregulation? *International Journal of Psychophysiology*, *13*(2), 97–100. https://doi.org/10.1016/0167-8760(92)90048-g

Ekor, M. (2014). The growing use of herbal medicines: issues relating to adverse reactions and challenges in monitoring safety. *Frontiers in Pharmacology*, *4*(177). https://doi.org/10.3389/fphar.2013.00177

Elizabeth, L., Machado, P., Zinöcker, M., Baker, P., & Lawrence, M. (2020). Ultra-Processed Foods and Health Outcomes: A Narrative Review. *Nutrients*, *12*(7), 1955. https://doi.org/10.3390/nu12071955

Fenton, T. R., Eliasziw, M., Lyon, A. W., Tough, S. C., & Hanley, D. A. (2008). Meta-analysis of the quantity of calcium excretion associated with the net acid excretion of the modern diet under the acid-ash diet hypothesis. *The American Journal of Clinical Nutrition*, *88*(4),

1159–1166.
https://doi.org/10.1093/ajcn/88.4.1159

Ferreira, M. (2020, August 17). *Sen Lines and Herbal Compresses | Sen Sip.* TraditionalBodywork.com. https://www.traditionalbodywork.com/herbal-compresses-and-the-sib-sen-energy-lines/

Genome. (2022). *Carcinogen.* Genome.gov. https://www.genome.gov/genetics-glossary/Carcinogen

Gitalis, J. (2018, September 6). *The Dark Side of White Salt.* Josh Gitalis. https://www.joshgitalis.com/the-dark-side-of-white-salt/

Grief Speaks. (2022). *Traumatic and Sudden Loss.* Griefspeaks.com. http://griefspeaks.com/id107.html

Groves, M. (2018, October 12). *12 Science-Backed Benefits of Peppermint Tea and Extracts.* Healthline. https://www.healthline.com/nutrition/pepperm int-tea#TOC_TITLE_HDR_2

Hafner, C. (2016). *Moxibustion | Taking Charge of Your Health & Wellbeing.* Taking Charge of Your Health & Wellbeing. https://www.takingcharge.csh.umn.edu/explor e-healing-practices/moxibustion

Haider, P. (2018, July 27). *6 Proven Health Benefits Of Banlangen Keli Tea.* Sivana East. https://blog.sivanaspirit.com/hh-proven-health-benefits-of-banlangen-keli-tea/

Haider, P. (2022). *"7 Proven Health Benefits of Banlangen Keli Tea."* Www.selfgrowth.com.

https://www.selfgrowth.com/articles/7-

proven-health-benefits-of-banlangen-keli-tea

Health Essentials. (2021, August 30). *What is Reiki, and Does it Really Work?* Cleveland Clinic. https://health.clevelandclinic.org/reiki/

Health Guide Info. (2010, December 19). *What Are the Harmful Effects of Spicy Food?* Www.healthguideinfo.com. https://www.healthguideinfo.com/nutrition-basics/p99958/

Healthline. (2018, June 3). *11 Reasons Why Too Much Sugar Is Bad for You*. Healthline. https://www.healthline.com/nutrition/too-much-sugar#TOC_TITLE_HDR_8

Healthschoolguide. (2022). *Aromatherapist | Education Requirements & Training Programs*. Www.healthschoolguide.net.

https://www.healthschoolguide.net/health-careers/how-to-become-an-aromatherapist/

HealthySupplementsGuide. (2022, March 13). *Do You Believe That Natural Supplements Make A Significant Difference?* Healthy Supplements Guide. https://www.healthysupplementsguide.com/2022/03/13/do-you-believe-that-natural-supplements-make-a-significant-difference/

Hitti, M. (2016, December 14). *What Is Traditional Chinese Medicine?* WebMD; WebMD. https://www.webmd.com/balance/guide/what-is-traditional-chinese-medicine

Homeopathic Medicine. (2020, August 21). *What is Homeopathic Medicine? #1 Natural Healing Remedies.* Homeopathicmedicine.one.

https://homeopathicmedicine.one/what-is-homeopathic-medicine/

Huffington Post. (2006, May 8). *Why People Get Sick.* HuffPost. https://www.huffpost.com/entry/why-people-get-sick_b_20599

Jackie. (2020, October 21). *Sedentary? That's Dangerous.* Somebodystrong. https://www.besomebodystrong.com/post/sedentary-that-s-dangerous

Jaiswal, Y. S., & Williams, L. L. (2017). A glimpse of Ayurveda – The forgotten history and principles of Indian traditional medicine. *Journal of Traditional and Complementary Medicine,* *7*(1), 50–53. https://doi.org/10.1016/j.jtcme.2016.02.002

Jeanroy, A. (2022, April 1). *Learn How to Make the Perfect Herbal Infusion at Home*. The Spruce Eats. https://www.thespruceeats.com/how-to-make-an-herbal-infusion-1762142

Jun 5, F. | H. 3471 | P., & Print, 2017 |. (2017). *Herb Infused Oils*. Home & Garden Information Center | Clemson University, South Carolina. https://hgic.clemson.edu/factsheet/herb-infused-oils/

Justis, A. (2016, October 5). *How to Make an Herbal Syrup*. Herbal Academy. https://theherbalacademy.com/herbal-syrup/

Kessler, D. M., & DC. (2018, May 16). *15 Amazing Health Benefits of Peppermint Tea*. Doctors Health Press - Daily Free Health Articles and Natural Health Advice. https://www.doctorshealthpress.com/general-health-articles/health-benefits-of-peppermint-tea/

Khazan, O. (2014, May 21). *How Being Poor Makes You Sick*. The Atlantic. https://www.theatlantic.com/health/archive/2014/05/poverty-makes-you-sick/371241/

Lad, V. (2021, August 25). *Introduction to Panchakarma*. Ayurveda. https://www.ayurveda.com/introduction-to-panchakarma/

Leung, C. W., Laraia, B. A., Needham, B. L., Rehkopf, D. H., Adler, N. E., Lin, J., Blackburn, E. H., & Epel, E. S. (2014). Soda and Cell Aging: Associations Between Sugar-Sweetened Beverage Consumption and Leukocyte Telomere Length in Healthy Adults From the National Health and

Nutrition Examination Surveys. *American Journal of Public Health*, *104*(12), 2425–2431. https://doi.org/10.2105/AJPH.2014.302151

Lin, H. D., & Gao, G. J. (2013). Transportation Safety Countermeasure Analysis on Cold-Chain Logistics of Fresh Agricultural Products. *Advanced Materials Research, 860-863*(8), 3123–3127. https://doi.org/10.4028/www.scientific.net/amr.860-863.3123

Lombardo, C. (2018, November 28). *Why is Yoga a Holistic Practice?* Celebrate Yoga. https://celebrateyoga.org/yoga-holistic-practice/

Louis, D. (2019). *Herbal Infused Oils: Uses & Benefits*. Intentional Theory.

https://intentionaltheory.com/blogs/news/uses-benefits-of-infused-herbal-oils

Mamgain, S. (2010, January 29). *Benefits of Herbalism.* EzineArticles. https://ezinearticles.com/?Benefits-of-Herbalism&id=3661226

Mantri, S. (2008). Holistic Medicine and the Western Medical Tradition. *AMA Journal of Ethics, 10*(3), 177–180. https://doi.org/10.1001/virtualmentor.2008.10.3.mhst1-0803.

Marks, H. (2011, March 2). *What Is Holistic Medicine?* WebMD; WebMD. https://www.webmd.com/balance/guide/what-is-holistic-medicine

Mayo Clinic. (2017). *Herbal supplements: What to know before you buy.* Mayo Clinic.

https://www.mayoclinic.org/healthy-lifestyle/nutrition-and-healthy-eating/in-depth/herbal-supplements/art-20046714

Mayo Clinic. (2018). *Acupuncture.* Mayoclinic.org. https://www.mayoclinic.org/tests-procedures/acupuncture/about/pac-20392763

McEvoy, M. (2020, December 14). *Organic 101: five steps to organic certification.* Www.usda.gov. https://www.usda.gov/media/blog/2012/10/10/organic-101-five-steps-organic-certification

Medicine World. (2022). *A short history of holistic medicine : Information from MedicineWorld.org.* Medicineworld.org. https://medicineworld.org/alternative/holistichealth/a-short-history-of-holistic-medicine.html

Megraoui, B. (2018, February 26). *What To Know About The 3 White Poisons: Flour, Sugar And*

Salt. Society19 UK. https://www.society19.com/uk/the-3-white-poisons-flour-sugar-and-salt/

Micozzi, M. S. (2006). *Fundamentals of Complementary and Integrative Medicine.* Saunders.

NANP. (2020, June 11). *What is Holistic Nutrition? | National Association of Nutrition Professionals.* NANP. https://nanp.org/what-is-holistic-nutrition/

Narayanaswamy, V. (1981). Origin and Development of Ayurveda: (A Brief History). *Ancient Science of Life, 1*(1), 1–7.

National Cancer Institute. (2021). *What Is Cancer?* National Cancer Institute; Cancer.gov. https://www.cancer.gov/about-cancer/understanding/what-is-cancer

National Institute of Environmental Health Sciences. (2018). *Air Pollution and Your Health.* National Institute of Environmental Health Sciences. https://www.niehs.nih.gov/health/topics/agents/air-pollution/index.cfm

National Qigong Association. (2022). *What is Qigong?* Www.nqa.org. https://www.nqa.org/what-is-qigong-

National Toxicology Program. (2022). *Traffic-related Air Pollution and Hypertensive Disorders of Pregnancy.* Ntp.niehs.nih.gov. https://ntp.niehs.nih.gov/whatwestudy/assessments/noncancer/completed/pollution/index.html

Natural Healers. (2016, October 7). *Read a History of Holistic Health & Its Evolution | Natural*

Healers. Natural Healers. https://www.naturalhealers.com/blog/holistic-health-history/

Non-GMO Project. (2016). *What is a GMO?* Nongmoproject.org; The Non-GMO project. https://www.nongmoproject.org/gmo-facts/what-is-gmo/

Nong, S. (2002). *Holistic Concept of Chinese Medicine.* Www.shen-Nong.com. http://www.shen-nong.com/eng/principles/holism.html

Noveille, A. (2015, April 24). *How To Make A Poultice With Dried & Fresh Herbs.* Herbal Academy. https://theherbalacademy.com/how-to-make-a-poultice-with-herbs/

O'Connor, A. (2008, June 17). The Claim: A Spicy Meal Before Bed Can Disrupt Sleep. *The New*

York *Times*. https://www.nytimes.com/2008/06/17/health/1 7real.html

Occhipinti, A. (2019). *8 Key Questions Holistic Nutrition Professionals Should Ask New Clients.* Afpafitness.com. https://www.afpafitness.com/blog/8-key-questions-holistic-nutrition-professionals-should-ask-new-clients

Okada, H., Kuhn, C., Feillet, H., & Bach, J.-F. . (2010). The "hygiene hypothesis" for autoimmune and allergic diseases: an update. *Clinical & Experimental Immunology, 160*(1), 1–9. https://doi.org/10.1111/j.1365-2249.2010.04139.x

Oumeish, O. Y. (1998). The Philosophical, Cultural, and Historical Aspects of Complementary,

Alternative, Unconventional, and Integrative Medicine in the Old World. *Archives of Dermatology*, *134*(11). https://doi.org/10.1001/archderm.134.11.1373

Pagidipati, N. J., & Gaziano, T. A. (2013). Estimating Deaths From Cardiovascular Disease: A Review of Global Methodologies of Mortality Measurement. *Circulation*, *127*(6), 749–756. https://doi.org/10.1161/circulationaha.112.128413

Parkin, E. (2019, June 1). *What Does a Kinesiologist Do? | InHome Physical Therapy | Edmonton & Calgary*. InHome Physical Therapy & Massage. https://www.inhomephysicaltherapy.ca/blog/what-does-a-kinesiologist-do/

Patterson, E. (2020, November 28). *What is Homeopathy? Which is the Best Homeopathy Hospital in India?* Fit Living Tips. https://www.fitlivingtips.com/best-homeopathy-hospital-in-india/

Penman, T. (2013, August 4). *How to Make an Herbal Decoction.* Holistic Health Herbalist. https://www.holistichealthherbalist.com/how-to-make-an-herbal-decoction/

Petre, A. (2018, December 17). *8 Health Benefits of Yerba Mate (Backed by Science).* Healthline. https://www.healthline.com/nutrition/8-benefits-of-yerba-mate#TOC_TITLE_HDR_9

Petre, A. (2020, July 9). *What Happens If You Eat Too Much Salt?* Healthline. https://www.healthline.com/nutrition/what-happens-if-you-eat-too-much-salt

Petri, R. P., Delgado, R. E., & McConnell, K. (2015). Historical and Cultural Perspectives on Integrative Medicine. *Medical Acupuncture*, *27*(5), 309–317. https://doi.org/10.1089/acu.2015.1120

Phillips, V. (2022). *Are Your Bed Sheets Making You Sick?* Www.refinery29.com. https://www.refinery29.com/en-us/2015/05/86717/dust-mites-bed-sheets-allergies-sick

Psychalive. (2009, June 7). *I Feel Lonely: What To Do When You're Feeling Alone.* PsychAlive. https://www.psychalive.org/isolation-and-loneliness/

Reiki Administrator. (2014, October 15). *What is Reiki?* Reiki. https://www.reiki.org/faqs/what-reiki

Repshealth. (2022). *Understanding Air Pollution.* Respiratory Health Association. https://resphealth.org/clean-air/understanding-air-pollution/#:~:text=levels%20are%20elevated.-

Ruggeri, C. (2021). *11 Best Herbal Tea Options.* Dr. Axe. https://draxe.com/nutrition/herbal-tea-benefits/

Safeopedia. (2022). *What is Toxic Gas? - Definition from Safeopedia.* Safeopedia.com. https://www.safeopedia.com/definition/2337/toxic-gas

Schwalfenberg, G. K. (2012). The Alkaline Diet: Is There Evidence That an Alkaline pH Diet Benefits Health? *Journal of Environmental and Public Health, 2012*(12), 1–7. https://doi.org/10.1155/2012/727630

Sissi Wachtel-Galor. (2011). *Herbal Medicine Biomolecular and Clinical Aspects, Second Edition*. Crc Press.

Smith Nicholson, C. (2020, February 25). *What is an Aromatherapist, Are They Certified & Should You Visit One?* Easy Essential Oils. https://easyessentialoils.co/certified-aromatherapist/

Son of China. (2021, September 27). *What Is Chinese Cupping Therapy And Does It Work? (Ba Guan)*. Sonofchina.com. https://sonofchina.com/china-traditions/what-is-cupping-in-chinese-medicine/

Sorrow, A. R. (2013, May 30). *UGA research uncovers cost of resiliency in kids*. UGA Today. https://news.uga.edu/uga-research-uncovers-cost-of-resiliency-in-kids/

src="https://secure.gravatar.com/avatar/78cb33b2ac7 43413a018a58549df3110?s=50, img class="avatar" alt="Abbey S., #038;d=mm, Jun. 24, 038;r=g" width="50" height="50">Abbey S., & 2021. (2022). *10 Things in Your House That Could Be Making You Sick.* The Healthy. https://www.thehealthy.com/home/your-messy-house-is-making-you-sick/

src="https://www.thehealthy.com/wp-content/uploads/2020/02/Emily-DiNuzzo-Headshot_The-Healthy.jpg?fit=50, img class="avatar" alt="Emily D., Jun. 11, 50" width="50" height="50">Emily D., & 2021. (2021, June 14). *How Often Should You Wash Your Sheets? Here's What Germ Experts Recommend.* The Healthy.

https://www.thehealthy.com/habits/how-often-you-should-wash-your-sheets/

Swee. (2019, August 16). *Bitterness and its side-effects on health.* Swee10-Blog. https://www.swee10.com/sweetblog/bitterness-and-its-side-effects-on-health/

Thapa, S., Fischbach, L. A., Delongchamp, R., Faramawi, M. F., & Orloff, M. (2019). Association between Dietary Salt Intake and Progression in the Gastric Precancerous Process. *Cancers, 11*(4), 467. https://doi.org/10.3390/cancers11040467

The Editors of Encyclopaedia Britannica. (2019). traditional Chinese medicine | Description, History, & Facts. In *Encyclopædia Britannica.* https://www.britannica.com/science/traditional-Chinese-medicine

Tian, S. (2010, September 29). *Advantages and Disadvantages of Herbal Medicine | HealthGuidance.* Healthguidance.org. https://www.healthguidance.org/entry/12415/1/advantages-and-disadvantages-of-herbal-medicine.html

Traditional Medicinals. (2020). *Herbal Basics: Tonics 101 - Traditional Medicinals - Herbal Wellness.* Traditional Medicinals. https://www.traditionalmedicinals.com/articles/plants/the-basics-herbal-tonics/

Trani, J.-F., & Bakhshi, P. (2013). Vulnerability and mental health in Afghanistan: Looking beyond war exposure. *Transcultural Psychiatry, 50*(1), 108–139. https://doi.org/10.1177/1363461512475025

University of Natural Health. (2019, July 29). *5 Advantages of Holistic Healing | University of Natural Health.* Naturalhealthcollege. https://naturalhealthcollege.org/5-advantages-of-holistic-healing/

US EPA. (2016, March 21). *What is ozone? | US EPA.* US EPA. https://www.epa.gov/ozone-pollution-and-your-patients-health/what-ozone

US EPA. (2018, November 14). *Particulate Matter (PM) Basics.* US EPA. https://www.epa.gov/pm-pollution/particulate-matter-pm-basics

VeryHealthyLife. (2019, January 7). *10 GMO Foods You Must Avoid Eating - Page 10 of 11.* Very Healthy Life. https://veryhealthy.life/10-gmo-foods-you-must-avoid-eating/10/

Verywellhealth. (2022). *How Common Is It to Have Both Anxiety and Depression?* Verywell Health. https://www.verywellhealth.com/depression-and-anxiety-signs-symptoms-and-treatment-5191284

Walter, S. (2019). *American Holistic Health Association.* American Holistic Health Association. https://ahha.org/selfhelp-articles/holistic-health/

Wilson, D. R. (2019, April 17). *Tuina Massage: Benefits, Techniques, and More.* Healthline. https://www.healthline.com/health/tuina#how-it-works

Yang, Y. (2010). *Decoction - an overview | ScienceDirect Topics.* Www.sciencedirect.com.

https://www.sciencedirect.com/topics/medicine-and-dentistry/decoction

Made in the USA
Monee, IL
27 July 2023

6a212eda-7d64-40a8-b54c-d2672686d2b2R02